Ageless Warrior Fitness

Anti-Aging, Health, and Fitness
by
Julio Anta

Edited by David R. Slentz

Cover Photo by Thomas Arnold

Anta's Fitness and Self Defense, Inc.

1

Disclaimer

The exercises and advice within this book may be too strenuous or dangerous for some people. The reader(s) should consult a physician before engaging in them.

The author is not a medical doctor or nutritionist. The book is based on the author's experience and what has worked for him.

The author and publisher of this book are not responsible in any manner whatsoever for any injury which may occur through reading and following the instructions herein.

Dedication

This book is dedicated to my father, Julio C. Anta, the hardest working man I've ever known. My dad was a rough and tough man's man. He led by example and taught me the greatest lesson: how to be a man. Your kids may not remember what you say; but they will remember what you do. Thank you, Dad, for leading the way.

I also dedicate this book to my incredible wife, Elena, and my two extraordinary boys, Julio and Jon-Paul and my newly born grandson Harold David Anta. Thank you for giving me the inspiration to write this book and for living life in the martial arts way of living fit and fearless.

Most of all, this book is dedicated to my Lord and Savior, Jesus Christ, who transformed my life and has blessed me with health and wisdom.

Contents

Chapter 3

Nutrition/Supplements

Chapter 4

Introduction

The Ageless Warrior Fitness is dedicated to everyone who wants to live life to the fullest at any age. It will inspire you and give you information on staying lean, fit and healthy in your 40's, 50's, 60's, and above. The Ageless Warrior philosophy is "Train like a 50-year-old and you'll look like a 50-year-old. Set no limitations. Train like an Ageless Warrior and you'll look like a warrior."

It is a life-changing guide for everyone who believes that the best is yet to come. It is also an encouragement for those poor souls that feel that their best years have passed and are long and gone. It doesn't matter if you were the star athlete in high school, or the last one picked. It doesn't matter if you are in your 30's or 100's. If you believe you can, then you can! You can achieve your goals. I can lead the way for you, but you must believe. The best is yet to come.

Following the Ageless Warrior fitness program will help you slow down the aging process. It will show you how to slow down or even reverse muscle loss which starts in your thirties. I was able to reverse it and I'm slowly building more muscle. The only time that I've been more muscular was between my mid-to-late twenties when I was a competitive bodybuilder. I am more muscular now than when I was a teen, in early twenties, thirties, forties, and even in my early fifties. Following my methods in this book will help speed up your metabolism to help you lose weight. It will improve your balance, flexibility and coordination.

This book is based on my experience, success and failures. This is not based on the theory or books of any fitness guru, personal trainer, overweight or anti-aging doctor. I'm not a doctor or anti-aging expert. I cannot prescribe a program for you. I'm just a person that has found how I can look young and stay fit and healthy. I train around my maladies and injuries. I've accomplish more in my fifties than ever before. I'm living life to the fullest. The Ageless Warrior is how, with trial and error, I discovered my own fountain of youth. I'm sure that there are other ways to stay fit and look younger than your biological age. The Ageless Warrior Fitness is just like the lyrics of Frank Sinatra's song "My Way." Yes, I did it my way and I found the answer to looking younger and staying fit while living fearless.

You've heard the cliché "Age is just a number"? I'm sure that you also have heard people as young as 30 years old say, "I can't do that. I'm not that young anymore." Or "When I was younger I could do that and more." So, who should you listen to? If age is just a number you should be able to accomplish most of your fitness goals at any age. Yet, as we age it is apparent that most people lose muscle tone, speed, endurance and flexibility. Yes, it is true that as we age, our body deteriorates. Our hormone level lowers, our metabolism slows down, and we lose flexibility, endurance and strength.

The key to staying in shape and looking young at any age is healthy living, consistency, training around injuries and believing you can. You need to eat healthy, stretch, do cardio and most important do progressive strength training so that we can delay and change the aging process. Staying away from smoking, alcohol and drugs is also very important. So, I do believe that age is just a number as long as you work out with wisdom and intensity. I strongly believe that at 57, if I think and workout like a 50-year-old, then I will look, feel and act like a 50-year-old. I train wisely to avoid injuries, yet I train hard and heavy, and do not put any limitations on what I can do or on my goal setting.

The worse enemy of anti-aging is lack of regular exercise. As you age and don't find the time to exercise, our bones weaken, we get flabbier, our joints hurt, muscles shrinks, skin sags and wrinkles, joints hurt, you tire easily, and end up with bad posture.

My wife tells me to stop telling people this story because they'll think that I'm crazy. Yet, we are all motivated to change things by different circumstances. So, here is one of the crazy reasons that I decided to build more muscle. When I first noticed the skin wrinkling under my elbow at age 49, I panicked and started doing research on anti-aging. That's when I decided to start working out harder and with heavier weight to build more muscle. My goal was to look muscular by the age of 50. Since then I've slowly made gains. After injuries and illness, I had to go back to the drawing board as the old saying goes. I strongly believe in the Japanese Proverb "Fall down seven times get up eight." Every year after the age of 49 I've looked better and am in much better shape.

I am a student for life and my goal is to lead you by example. The goal of this book is to teach you the way to strength, health, fitness, and looking and feeling younger. Through nutrition and proper exercise we can slow down the hand of time.

I believe that you should always lead by example. I learn this as a young adult at Marine Corps Recruit Training Center, better known at boot camp, in Parris Island, South Carolina. Parris Island is also known as the land that God forgot. While in boot camp your drill instructors expect a lot from you physically and mentally, yet they lead by example and will outdo the recruits in every endeavor. Everything that I write and recommend in The Ageless Warrior I am currently doing or have done in the past.

One of my pet peeves is the anti-aging and fitness expert or gurus that don't look the part. I believe that if you are going to listen to an anti-aging fitness expert he or she must look the part. They should look healthy, fit, younger than their age and muscular. Why would anyone in their right mind follow a fitness instructor that doesn't look healthy, strong and young? Most people expect someone over 40 to not look muscular or strong. That is a fallacy. You can slow down the aging process to look young, be healthy, strong and fit at any age.

If you are not satisfied with the way you look you can change. Don't let anyone tell you that you are too old or too far out of shape. If you are not in the shape that I'm in, you might ask yourself, "Can I do it?" Can I look like him even though I haven't exercised in 30 years? Sure you can if you are persistent and go on a safe workout routine geared for longevity. Now, if I want to look like Sly Stallone who is 10 1/2 years older than me, could I? You might say, "No, I can't." Sly has chefs to cook his healthy meals, nutritionist, personal trainers and coaches on his staff and the best home gym and equipment in the world. Yet, my answer to that same question is, "Sure I can!" If I believe I can, work out hard, do more cardio, and eat healthier, then I can be built even better than Sly. Remember Henry Ford's quote "Whether you think you can, or you think you can't – you're right."

I remember in my early 40's looking at fitness books at the local bookstore for over-40-year-olds and seniors. To my surprise, all the books I saw were using models that looked old, had gray hair and no muscle tone at all. What was worse was that they were using 10 and 15 pound dumbbells. I can totally understand a sedentary senior or someone going through rehab after an injury using such light weights, yet how can a healthy normal 40-year-old workout with such little intensity or goals? The problem here is that the old-looking, weak senior in the book is the norm and expectation. What most trainers and books teach on training for those over the age of 40 is erroneous. They have the client doing long low intensity cardio and light weights. To turn the hands of time you must workout with heavy weight. Heavy weight training increases testosterone. At 57 years old, I am proof that you can be healthy and gain muscles at any age.

There is an old joke in the martial arts industry that says that the higher the degree on the black belt, the bigger the belly and the smaller the tip of the black belt becomes. They call themselves masters, yet they have not mastered their own life. I want to help you change your life by teaching you how to master your health and fitness. The Ageless Warrior will also help you train around injuries and illness.

At my martial arts/fitness center, all instructors are required to be in shape and look the part from my youngest instructor my son Jon-Paul who is 19 (as I write this) to all other instructors who are in their 40's, and even to me at 57.

The only time that I looked better than I do today was in my late 20's when I was a competitive bodybuilder. I look better today at 57 than in my teens, early 20's, 30's, 40's and early 50's. Even though I have numerous injuries, overall I'm in the best shape of my life. My goal with God's blessing is to be in the best shape of my life and for my body to look better than ever at age 60.

I stopped competitive bodybuilding after dislocating both shoulders sparring at a karate tournament at age 28. I was told by doctors that I would never be able to lift weights or do martial arts again. This was the biggest shock of my life. I had been doing martial arts on and off since I was 13 and serious bodybuilding since I was 18.

Let me give you an overview of some of the things I've accomplished at an age when most people have stopped setting goals. These goals were accomplished going around and struggling with numerous injuries.

At 29, after the shoulder injuries, I gave my life to Christ and met my future wife in church.

In my 30's, I continued studying different martial arts, got married, started a new career as a corrections officer, my two sons were born, and I won numerous trophies in kung fu and karate tournaments while studying kung fu.

At 40, I earned a black sash (belt) in Hung Gar Kung Fu. At 41 I opened Anta's Fitness and Self Defense and was certified in Kardio Karate. At 43, I retired from the Department of Corrections to become a full-time martial arts instructor. While in my 40's, I grew my school into one of the largest martial arts schools in South Florida and the largest in Doral. I became NAPMA's Spanish representative and later its Florida director. I was a speaker in three NAPMA World conferences. NAPMA at that time was the first and largest martial arts industry organization. We were featured in numerous TV shows, newspapers and magazines

In my 50's, I was certified as an instructor in Jeet Kune Do, Krav Maga, and Muay Thai Kickboxing. I was certified in kettlebells with various organizations, Battling Ropes, Indian clubs, Action Strength, Elite Combat Fitness, and MMA Fighter Fit.

On June 9, 2014, at 57 years old, I was promoted to blue belt in Gracie Jiu Jitsu under the Valenti Brothers. This was special because I tried studying Brazilian Jiu Jitsu at different times in my life and got injured right away. At one time I started to believe that I could never do Jiu Jitsu due to reoccurring injuries while training. My friend, Alfred Magnan, told me that the Valenti Brothers trained you in a safe environment for longevity. When they opened a branch in Coral Gables I joined the school. I have two amazing instructors, Burak Eyilik and Jimmy Robertson. Now I'm hooked to study Gracie Jiu Jitsu for a lifetime. Never say never. Where there's a will, there's a way.

My claim to fame and what I'm mostly known for is for my martial arts success. I run one of the most successful martial arts training centers in Florida. Since I started teaching martial arts 16 years ago in 1998, I have been featured in over 150 TV shows. In 2013, I appeared in nineteen TV shows mostly for Anti-Bullying, Child Safety, and Women Self-Defense. I have authored two videos "Anta's Art of Fighting Without Fighting Anti-Bullying" and "Anta's Shaolin Physical Conditioning."

I believe that my biggest accomplishment and expertise is in fitness, but especially in senior fitness. Most people are amazed that I'm in my late 50's. I'm usually told that I look like I was in my early 40's.

Just recently I found a motivational video on Facebook of Arnold Schwarzenegger talking about his 6 Rules for Success.
1. Trust Yourself
2. Break the Rules
3. Don't be Afraid
4. Ignore the Naysayers
5. Work Like Hell
6. Give Something Back

I have admired Arnold since the 1970's when I first started bodybuilding. I've followed his career as a competitive bodybuilder to becoming a movie star and even to becoming a politician. He set high goals and achieving them. He is arguably the greatest bodybuilder, a top action hero of the silver screen and became the governor of California. The most interesting part of this is that even though I never put together these six principles, I have been following them for many years. I pretty much said it in a different way: believe in myself, I did it my way, never give up, stay away from negative people, protect my inner circle, work while my competition is sleeping, tithe to my church, and help others achieve their goals.

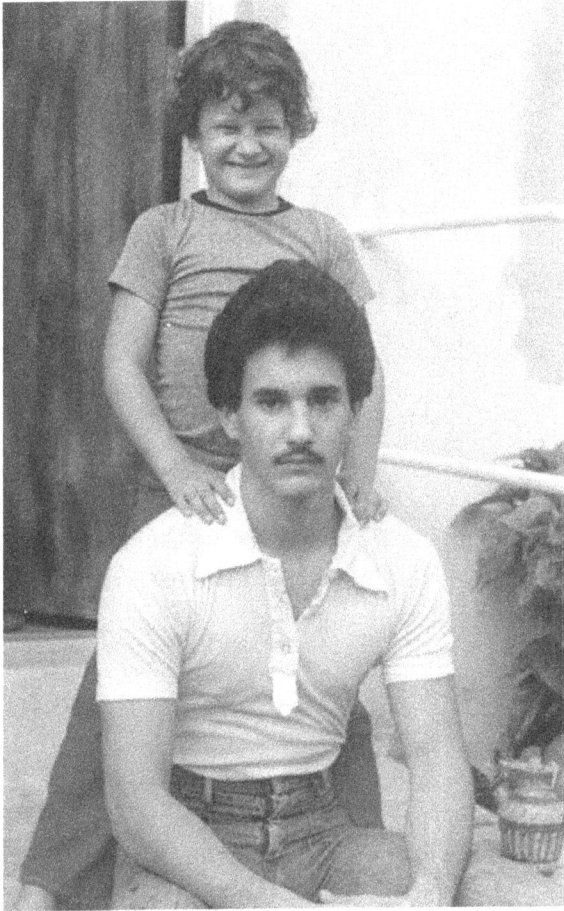

With my little brother Peter in 1975 or   1976
started bodybuilding with 11 or 12 inch arms

The Ageless Warrior is for everyone that is looking to set goals in order to stay strong, healthy and fit as they grow older. It is my personal journey to find my personal fountain of youth. Yes, age is just a number.

Chapter 1
Ageless Warrior

"Train like a 50-year-old
and you'll look like a 50-year-old.
Set no limitations.
Train like an Ageless Warrior
and you'll look like an Ageless Warrior!"

Julio Anta

What is an Ageless Warrior?

What is an Ageless Warrior? No, it's not like the fictional classical novel the "Portrait of Dorian Grey." In this classic story, Dorian sold his soul to the devil and only a painting of his portrait aged. Nor is an Ageless Warrior like the immortals in the movie and TV series "Highlander" that never aged. The Ageless Warrior is more like the Israeli Biblical hero, Caleb. Caleb was a spy and great warrior from the tribe of Judah. Caleb was a man of great faith and was allotted land and villages in the vicinity of Hebron. By this time he was 85 years of age and he was as strong as he had been a generation earlier when he first traveled through Canaan as a spy. He proved his strength and power by driving out the inhabitants. Caleb was a true Ageless Warrior. With healthy eating and physical training you too can be an Ageless Warrior. An Ageless Warrior is an attitude of success and never giving up, an attitude that will not use age as a crutch or an excuse. An Ageless Warrior is a person with a warrior's attitude that regardless of age, injuries or circumstances will strive to achieve their goals. You can be an Ageless Warrior.

This book is dedicated to the modern day Caleb's, the Ageless Warriors. Today the world has heard of numerous Ageless Warriors. We have role models such as Jack LaLanne the fitness guru who died at 97 and lived fit and fearless. Helio Gracie lived to be 95 years old and changed the martial arts world. Jhon Rhee the father of American Tae Kwon Do who is super fit. Rhee's philosophy is having the wisdom of 100 years with the body of a 20 year old. Vladimir Putin, president of Russia who at the age of 61 trains with heavy weights and is a martial artist. Putin published author of a book on Judo. Let's not forget Sly Stallone, star and writer of the Rocky movies. Today, he is 68 and is in better shape than ever. How about Chuck Norris in his 70's?

Going back further into history, we have numerous examples of Ageless Warriors. Joseph Pilates (1883-1967) lived to be 85 and is especially popular today as the creator of what we refer to as Pilates. Sig Klein (1902-1987) was a bodybuilder, weightlifter, strongman, writer, and gym operator. Klein was an ageless wonder posing and doing strongmen acts in his sixties. Who can forget Charles Atlas (1893-1972), the "World's Most Perfectly Developed Man" that created the Dynamic Tension Bodybuilding system. He proved that exercise and health paid off by staying fit until his death at the age of 80.

Being an Ageless Warrior is not just for men. Suzanne Summers of "Who's Company" is 68 and looks incredible. She is an anti-aging expert and has written numbers books on the

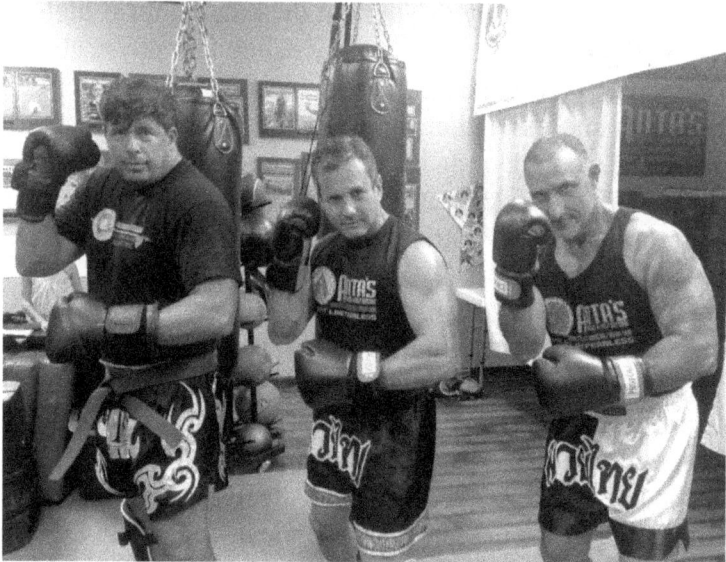

With my Ageless Warrior students Mike Catala 48 years old and Pedro Martinez 55 years old

subject. Christy Brinkley looks amazing at 60 and was on the cover of People magazine in a swim suit. How about Raquel Welsh who at 74, can wear a bikini and still look better than most women half her age. Do you know that Sofia Vergara is 41, Jennifer Aniston is 45, Cindy Crawford is 45, Nicole Kidman is 46, Salma Hayak is 47, Sandra Bullock is 50, Courtney Cox is also 50, and Demi Moore is 52? These leading ladies of Hollywood are still beautiful and fit women.

You might say, "Oh that's fine because they are celebrities who have chefs and nutritionists to fix them healthy meals, and they have personal trainers, and most likely they have even had plastic surgery. I'm just a normal person." Well, I'm just an ordinary person myself. I'm not a celebrity or a professional athlete. I don't have a personal chef, nutritionist,

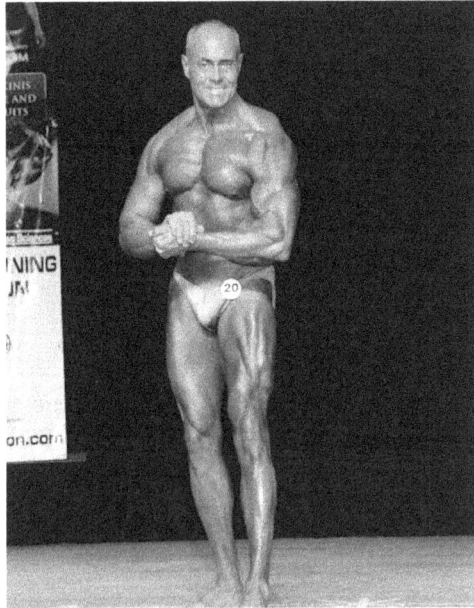

Lazaro Diaz 57 years old Bodybuilder multi title winner. Laz and I competed in the 1983 Miami Bodybuilding Champions

personal trainer, and neither have I had any plastic surgery. If I can do it, you can do it. I want to be your role model, leading you to become an Ageless Warrior just like Caleb. Stay fit for life by becoming an Ageless Warrior and defying the odds.

Think and train like a 50-year-old and you'll look and feel like a 50-year-old. Train like an Ageless Warrior and you'll look and feel like a warrior. Train without limitations.

The Ageless Warrior Fitness goal is to change your life. Everyone has that warrior spirit inside of them waiting to be awakened by the Ageless Warrior Fitness program.

Ageless Warrior Lifestyle

To live life to the fullest as an Ageless Warrior, you must change your lifestyle to take back your health and youth. It's not about diet and starting a fitness or martial arts program. It's about changing your lifestyle. The Bible says in Romans: "Do not conform to the pattern of this world, but be transformed by the renewing of your mind. Then you will be able to test and approve what God's will is –his good, pleasing and perfect will" (Romans 12:2, NIV).

First, it starts with discipline but with time it becomes a lifestyle. As I write this book, I've trained five days of weight

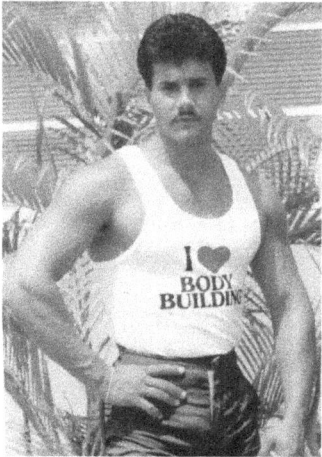

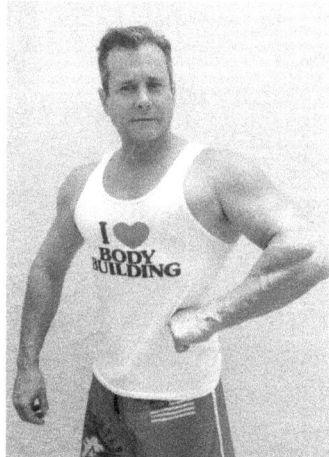

27 years old in 1984   30 years later   57 years old in 2014

training, four days Gracie Jiu Jitsu classes, two boxing classes, and I've taught numerous martial arts classes at my training center in this week alone. Am I tired? Sure I am, but I love it and would not change it for the world. I hate missing workouts. I feel that I'm blessed to have the health and endurance to do this type of training at age of 57.

STIC has a song by the name of "Warrior's Codes" in their album "The Workout." In the lyrics it says, "The Warrior lives

20

to train, The Warrior trains to live. The Warrior's code builds spirit, body, and mind." That to me is what the Ageless Warrior Fitness Lifestyle is all about. We train to live and live to train for longevity.

This week I was having a conversation with my Gracie Jiu Jitsu instructor, Jimmy Robertson of Valente Brothers Jiu Jitsu. Jimmy, a black belt with the rank of professor in Gracie Jiu Jitsu, does functional training and boxes. He was telling me that he is addicted to the rush of working out. I feel that this is the only addiction that is worth having. That is the Ageless Warrior Lifestyle. To an ancient warrior, his fighting skills and fitness was a matter of life or death.

The Ageless Warrior Fitness will help you start your journey to change your lifestyle on living a life of self-discipline, self-control and self-awareness. It's about winning over yourself to live the youthful life that you could only dream of.

I believe that it is sad that as children we dream of achieving great things, yet as we grow older due to responsibility, failure and hardship we forget our dreams. You can be the person you always wanted to be at any age. The answer is changing your lifestyle to an Ageless Warrior's fitness lifestyle. This will enable you to acquire physical and mental strength to achieve your goals and defy the aging process.

Each decade of my life has been memorable. Yet, reaching the half century has been amazing. I see life as a journey each decade as I set new goals. Looking forward to my 60's with God's help I'll be in better shape, a better martial artist, instructor, wiser and more successful. I'm sure that the best is yet to come. I will continue to live fit, fearless, and fabulous at 50 and beyond.

Recently at the gym, I was talking to Teo Hernandez who is 46 years old. He is a friend, personal trainer and firearms instructor. We were talking about a similar back injury we both had yet we were training. [Teo almost died in a hit-and-run accident while he was cycling a few years ago. He went from being super fit and strong to spending months in a hospital and having to undergo spinal surgery. Today he is back and in great shape!] I was telling Teo, saying, "If you train like a 50-year-old you will look like a 50-year-old." Teo later came to tell me that the guy he was training said this to him when I left, "Wow! He is 57, but he looks 40. That's 17 years younger." Now, I really do not think that I look 40 yet, but that sure is a great compliment. That's what Ageless Warrior training is all about: defying age.

One of the setbacks I've noticed in older martial arts instructors is the close-mindedness of believing that they know everything and have nothing to learn mentally or physically. Yet, as I mentioned earlier the older they get and the higher the degree on their black belt, the shorter their belt becomes due to the size of their belly. I believe that I'm a student for life. I learned this concept from my Haganah F.I.G.H.T (Fierce Israeli Guerrilla Hand to hand Tactics) instructor Mike Lee Kanarak. As a student for life I am constantly researching, studying and learning. I'm on a never-ending quest to develop my mind and body.

As I was finishing this book, I found out that my local chamber of commerce, the Doral Chamber of Commerce, was hosting a book self-publishing workshop by the chamber's president, Manny Sarmiento. I didn't think twice and signed up for the course. This made finishing and publishing this book so much easier. I am a student for life because knowledge is power.

Let me give you a quote from Tien T'ai which my Jeet Kune Do instructor Harinder Singh Sabharwal shared with me, "Given enough time, any man may master the physical. With enough knowledge, any man may become wise, but it is a true warrior who can master both, and surpass the result!"

My Life Story

From Charlie Brown to Superman

This is my story. I jokingly tell people that this is the title of my life story: "How Charlie Brown Grew Up to Become Superman!" As a child I was unpopular, didn't get good grades, and was the last one picked in physical education class. As an adult I was a Sergeant in the United States Marine Corps Reserves and a Corrections Officer. As an athlete, I've competed in Bodybuilding, Judo, Karate, Tae Kwon Do, Kung Fu, 5K and Dragon Boat Racing. My greatest success has come after the age of 50.

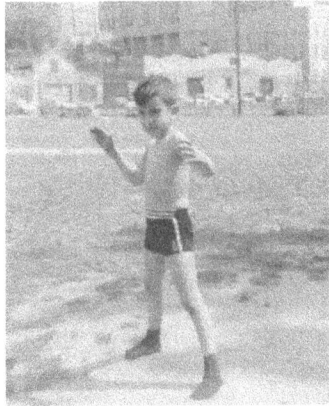

I was born in Cuba on April 29, 1957, a month premature. From a young age I was weak and sick. While still living in Cuba, I had to get an emergency appendix operation.

Fleeing an oppressive communist government, we flew from Cuba to Miami on April 2, 1962, which was 27 days before my fifth birthday. A few months later we moved to Yonkers, New York. We had to move for my father to be able to find work.

My love for bodybuilding and strength started as a young boy living in New York. One day as I was walking with my father to the house of my cousins, the Monserrat's, I noticed some photos of bodybuilders lying on the ground. Most likely, it was information on a bodybuilding course. I told my dad that I wanted to look like that when I grew up. He let me pick up the photos and take them with me.

I also remember watching Hercules on TV. In New York there was a channel that played the same movie for a full week. They were playing a Hercules movie starring Steve Reeves, Mr. America 1947, and Mr. Universe 1950. I watched it every day for the entire week. Some of our neighbors and friends thought that it was quite weird that this young boy was so obsessed with physical culture. At that time, fitness and bodybuilding were not very popular. When friends of my family would come to visit our home and I was watching Hercules, they would ask if they could change the channel. My dad fully supported me. He told them how much I loved that movie and that I should be allowed to continue watching it as much as I wanted. Even though I was skinny, sick, and weak, I was also a dreamer and prayed that one day I would look like Hercules. I will always be grateful and thank to my dad for supporting my crazy bodybuilding dreams. Steve Reeves has always been my favorite bodybuilder. My obsession with strength and manliness continued to grow. My parents would give me money and I would go buy comic books. I fantasized of being a super hero. They were muscular and helped those in need. I watched a lot of TV after school, but my favorite shows were those with the super heroes, Tarzan and Sons of Hercules TV series. I also loved watching WWF Wrestling in New York. I was truly a dreamer. I daydreamed becoming a movie star, super hero, wrestler, baseball player, military man, police officer, artist, black belt and bodybuilder.

My love for Martial Arts also began in New York at an early age. My first encounter with the martial arts was while watching a cartoon series.. I think this might have been Tom and Jerry. The mouse was dressed in a Gi (karate/judo uniform). The little mouse beat the cat by flipping him. I asked my dad to tell me what that mouse was doing to defeat such a big cat. My father told me that he was doing judo. Wow, this skinny, sickly boy that would fight a lot to defend against bullies even though did not like to fight finally found the answer to his problems. I told my dad I wanted to do judo. I did not study martial arts until I was in Jr High.

In 1966, the Green Hornet TV series aired. I loved it. I wanted to be just like Kato. I truly became a Bruce Lee fan in the 1970's when I saw his movie and the Kung Fu Mania began. It took me a while to discover that Lee was Kato and I had actually been his fan ever since the 1960's.

While living in New York I was very sick. I was given a penicillin vaccine and went into anaphylactic shock. I was even allergic to cold weather. In the winter time I had to take shots to survive. My allergist advised my parents that the best therapy for my allergies was going to the beach and sunbathing. He suggested that we move to Florida or to southern California. In 1966, we moved back to Miami Beach due to my numerous allergies.

In the summer of 1969, my parents bought a house in a suburb of Miami called Virginia Gardens. While living in Virginia Gardens, I started playing catch football in the street and would play basketball in the park. Believe it or not, I was 12 years old and had never ridden a bicycle. I finally learned to ride a bicycle that summer. I was still a terrible athlete, but at least I was very active.

For Christmas in 8th grade I asked for karate lessons. Karate was hard to find in 1972. My parents found a judo school in Hialeah, a neighboring city of Virginia Gardens. Within a few months I was promoted to yellow belt and I competed in my first judo tournament. To everyone's surprise, I won a trophy for third place. Due to peer pressure, I quit judo, the first sport that I had ever excelled in. I continue living with a very low self-esteem and I was extremely shy.

By the time I started high school, I started and quit at numerous karate schools. My brother, Mannie, was just the opposite of me. He is 3½ years younger than I am. He was very popular and an excellent athlete. When we started doing Kenpo Karate, I quit after a month, but Mannie became one of instructor Manny Reyes' top students. He later shined in both boxing and gymnastics.

During that time I had been reading bodybuilding magazines and wanted to look like Arnold, Franco Columbo, Serge Nubret, Dave Draper, Sergio Oliva, Frank Zane and the rest of the Muscle Beach guys of the seventies. My father bought me a plastic weight set and built a wooden incline bench for me. Finally, one summer, I began weight-lifting. Looking at my old photos today, it is obvious that I was starting to make gains. Sadly, though, by the beginning of that school year, I had stopped and was reverting back to my skinny, weak-looking self.

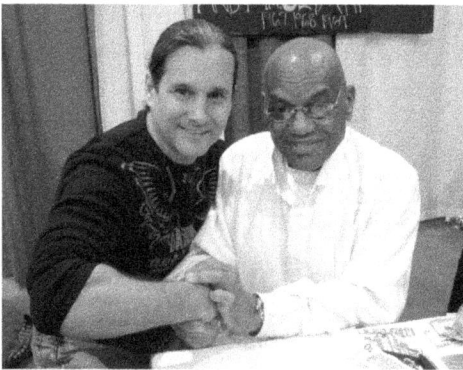

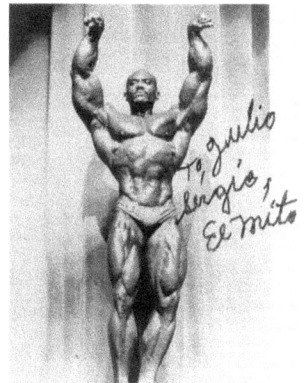

In 2008 with 3X Mr. Olympia Sergio Oliva "The Myth" who competed unit he was 44

It was in 1975, during my senior year that I first noticed a kid in our high school that was 6' 5" with 18 inch arms. His name was Mario Ramil. Apparently he had been going to Miami Springs Senior High ever since I started there, but I had never noticed him until then. Even though I was shy, I managed to ask him to help me start a workout. He refused, but I continued to hunt him down in order to ask for his help. In January of 1976, he assisted me in a workout and introduced me to another kid that was in my homeroom class at school. This kid was working out in Miami's first hardcore bodybuilding gym, Brodie's Gym. At the age of 18 ½, I started working out with him at Brodie's Gym and there was no turning back. Now, in 1976, all my friends were bodybuilders. To my surprise, I was

26

faster and doing better in my physical education class at school.

One day, Mario told me and some of my new bodybuilding buddies that he had met Jorge Navarrete, the current Mr. Florida. Navarrete was only 20 years old and he was the most impressive human being that I had ever seen. Jorge went on to win the Mr. North America and his height class in the Mr. America competition. One year later, Jorge started working at Brodie's Gym. He told me that I needed to train my shoulders and build them wider before I became 21. He said that after the age of 21, you could only build muscle on your shoulders, but not width. I will always be thankful to Jorge Navarrete for teaching me how to build large wide shoulders.

After high school I continued working out with Mario Ramil. By now he had 19 inch arms and we had become best friends. All of my friends were bodybuilders. My life revolved around training and going to the beach. Bodybuilding helped my self-esteem, yet I still remained extremely shy. While I was attending Miami-Dade College my dream came true. I started working at the college gym. There I met a high school kid that was called Muscles. He had the most incredible peak on his biceps, a tiny wasp-like waist with incredible abdominals. We became close friends and training partners. Mario and Muscles were my two biggest inspirations to train and build large muscles.

I started going to bodybuilding competitions. At one bodybuilding show, I was amazed to see great looking bodies even in the over-35-year-old division. From there on I said to myself that I would look like that as I aged gracefully.

In December 1980, at the age of 23, to the surprise of my bodybuilding friends and family, I fulfilled yet another childhood dream by joining the United Marine Corps Reserves. I lost much muscle in boot camp, but I was a proud U.S. Marine. After I got back to Miami, I continued to work out while in the Marine Corps Reserves. At the reserve center, things were so much different than in high school. I was popular among the Marines. I was now a muscular bodybuilder and admired by my fellow Marines.

How things started to change at that point in my life. This shy boy was now a popular, muscular Marine. Around 1983, I was promoted to sergeant. That same year I placed third in the Mr. Jr. Florida and at the Mr. Miami bodybuilding competition. Life was good. As a kid, I had associated myself with Charlie Brown, but now I felt like Superman. I even wore a gold chain with a Superman symbol.

At this point, I was becoming bigger and even more muscular, but life can change in minutes. Just one year later, I was diagnosed with hepatitis. By the time I recuperated, I had lost

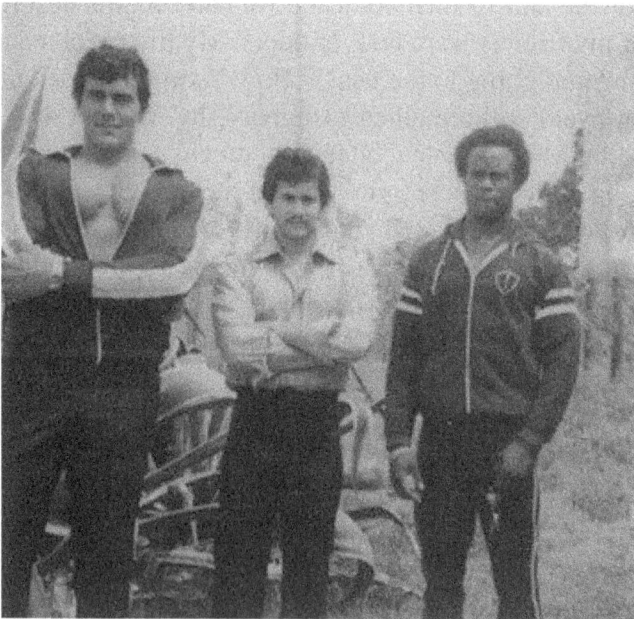

With my training partners Mario Ramil and Edward "Muscles" Hearns

over thirty pounds of muscle. By 1985, I had rebuilt my body and began competing again.

People were amazed with my transformation. I started a bodybuilding and martial arts act with my best friend, John Mandri. Our shows were choreographed with music from the current disco hits with bodybuilders and dancers performing in costumes. We performed in clubs in Miami, Ft. Lauderdale, and even at the College National Bodybuilding Championships. This reopened my appetite for martial arts. I continued bodybuilding, but also started studying karate. While competing in a karate tournament, I dislocated my shoulder. I continued to fight with my other arm, but then I also dislocated my other shoulder. Doctors told me not to work out or do any martial arts since it would only cause my shoulders to become worse. This was the end of my competitive bodybuilder career.

In 1986 I was depressed and started to go to church. God had bigger and better things for my life. I met my future wife, Elena, in church. I continued to study various kinds of martial arts and worked out with weights, even though, due to my injuries, I could not lift as intensely or heavily as I did in my competitive bodybuilding days. In September of 1990, I was hired to work at a maximum security prison, the South Florida Reception Center. In 1997, at the age of 40, I was promoted to black belt in Hung Gar Kung Fu. In 1998, while still working at the prison, I began teaching martial arts and fitness kickboxing. I started a new career at when I was 41. I worked at the prison for 10 years until 2000. It was in 2000 that I became a full-time martial arts and fitness professional.

In 1990, my first son, Julio III, was born. We made sure that he ate healthy, practiced martial arts, and participated in sports. In 1995, our second son, Jon-Paul, was born. We raised him the same as Julio. My wife, Elena, also raised our kids by example. She works out and is also quite fit. She used to teach Fitness Kickboxing and is currently teaching Pilates and Piloxing at our martial arts fitness center. She is certified as a level 2 instructor in MMA Fighter Fit. Health and fitness is a very important part of the Anta Family. We have raised two physically fit boys and we are leaving a fitness legacy in our family.

In the last 17 years, after receiving my first black belt, I continued my studies in other martial arts. I have been certified in Haganah F.I.G.H.T, Muay Thai, Jeet Kune Do and Krav Maga. In June 2014, I was promoted to blue belt in Gracie Jiu Jitsu. I have also been certified in kettlebells with three different organizations, in Battling ropes, Indian clubs, MMA Fighter Fit, Elite Combat Fitness, Youth Fitness Specialist, in Action Strength and as a personal trainer.

Today at 57 years old, I am in far better shape than ever, except for the time in my mid- to late 20's when I was competing. My goal is to be in better shape in my sixties than I was in my 30's, 40's, and 50's. As you can see from my story, most everything I've done in my life was to prepare me for a career in martial arts and fitness. Now, if I was able to change and succeed, my goal is to help you become an Ageless Warrior, defying the odds and helping you become fit and fearless for life.

I would like to thank God for how He has helped me in achieving my goals and living my childhood dreams of becoming a martial artist and bodybuilder. Today I live a great life as a martial arts and fitness professional. I praise God for transforming my life from an underachiever to a life of success, abundance, health and fitness. Most people just assume that I had been the popular jock in school, but the truth just the opposite. As a child, I associated myself with and actually felt just like Charlie Brown, yet I dreamed about one day being like Superman. Today, at 57, I am far closer to being like Superman (an Ageless Warrior, as I call it) than being like Charlie Brown.

You're Never Too Old to Start

I'm on a mission to get Americans, and especially older adults, fit and fearless by changing their mindset. I believe that not only you can increase your life expectancy, but better yet, you can increase the quality of your life by the actions you take. I know things do not become any easier as we grow older. When we age, it is true that we begin losing strength, endurance, flexibility, balance, etc. The list can go on and on, but there is good news! That aging process only happens because we stop moving, stop eating healthy, stop exercising enough and because we don't take the supplements we need. The good news is that everyone can improve and succeed regardless of what fitness level you are in. You are never too late or too old to start!

It's never too late to get into shape, start a new career, or to succeed. Most people in their later years are discouraged or afraid to try new things. You might have tried and failed in your younger years and feel that it is too late. You'll be surprised how many recognized names and celebrities were not discovered or achieved success until their later year.

You can say I was late bloomer. The older I get, the more I have succeeded. I started doing martial arts at 13, but did not get my black belt until I was 40. I was very inconsistent in my training. I did not start training consistently until 1989 when I was 32. I started taking Tae Kwon Do. I took a few months off when I was hired by the department of corrections and attended the academy. After the academy, I went back to my Tae Kwon Do training and earned my green belt. At the test I broke my toe and had to take some time off.

After that, my old bodybuilding partner and coach who was also now working as a corrections officer for Miami-Dade County, Joaquin Travesio (AKA Joe Travie), told me that he was studying karate at the academy which was at Miami-Dade College. I started studying Sansei Goju Ryu Karate under Ed Preston who was the head of the Police academy defensive

31

tactics department. I studied a full year with Preston. While studying Goju Ryu in 1992, I bumped into my kung fu instructor from the 1970's. I began studying Hung Gar Kung Fu at his house. Six months later in 1993 he opened a storefront school in Westchester. By 1997, at age 40, I earned the rank of black belt. This is an age when most people feel that their best years are behind. Seven months later at 41, I continued working for the State of Florida Department of Corrections and started teaching kung fu to kids and fitness kickboxing to adults. Two years later, I retired from the Department of Corrections and became a full time martial arts professional. Today I live the American dream, success and happiness. I can truly tell you that most people I've seen are not that happy with their job or career, but I sure am. I love changing lives through martial arts and fitness. I love Mondays because I get to train and workout in the morning and in the evening teach classes to change lives.

Believe me you can start a new career or a hobby and transform your body at any age. Here is a list of celebrities in their 30's to 70's that changed their lives at a later than usual age. Celebrities who became famous in their 30's: The famous opera singer, Andrea Bocelli, was not discovered until he was 34. What's more interesting is that at age 12 due to a soccer accident he was blind. The comedian Phyllis Dillard was 37 when by the time she was discovered.

Samuel L. Jackson had done some small roles before but did not become famous until he was 40 in Spike Lee's 1991 film Jungle Fever. Martial artist, Steven Seagal, was 40 years old when he became a star after his first movie, *Under Siege*, became a box office hit. In 1948 Soichiro Honda was 42 years old when he formed the Honda Motor Company and created the motorcycle. Marvel Comics, Stan Lee, did not succeed until he was 43 and Jack Kirby at 44. Julia Childs was almost 40 when she started cooking, 41 when she wrote her first book, and did not have her TV show until she was 51.

Dr. Ruth Westheimer became a household name at the age of 53, as a sex expert. Henry Ford introduced the Model T Ford automobile when he was 45 years old. At 60 years old, he created the first car assembly line.

Oscar Swahn was 60 when he won his first gold medal. He won two goal medals that year in deer shooting in 1912. In 1920, at 72 he won a silver medal making him the oldest winning Olympian. Colonel Sanders (Harlan David Sanders) was 65 years old when he started Kentucky Fried Chicken, yet prior to that he had been living in his car.

Grandma Moses began painting at 75. She was 76 when she finished her first painting. She lived another 25 years as a painter. She started selling her paintings for $3, yet lived to see them go for over $10,000.

I remember a quote by George Elliot which said, "It is never too late to be what you might have been."

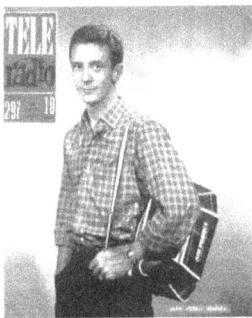

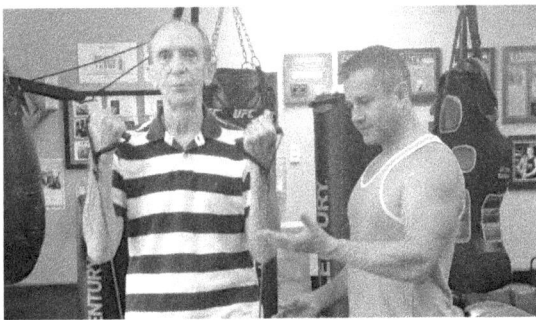

Cover of Spain's TV Guide   Juan Pedro Samoza training at 75 years old

Juan Pedro Samoza who was a famous actor, singer and director in Spain came to me because he was very weak and could not gain wait. He had never worked out in his life. Within a month and a half of training with me he gain 6 pounds. He also saw the shape of his deltoids and triceps. Samoza is now living the Ageless Warrior Lifestyle.

The Metamorphosis

Anta's Physical Transformation Timeline in Photos

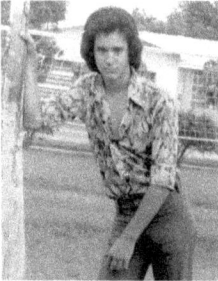
17 years old 115 pounds

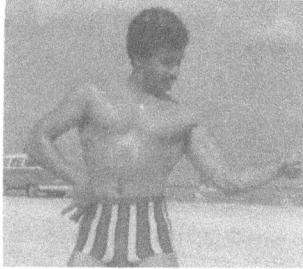
1st bodybuilding photo at 20

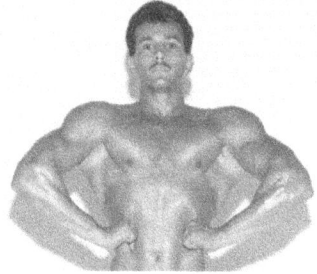
Competing at 26

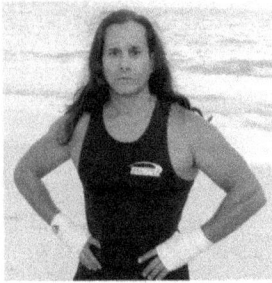
49 years old

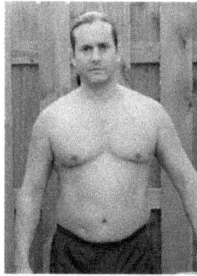
50 years old after injury

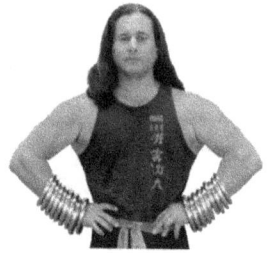
50 years old

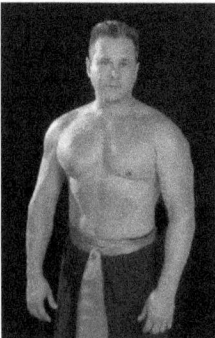
54 years old

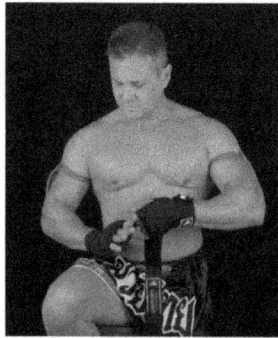
56 years old

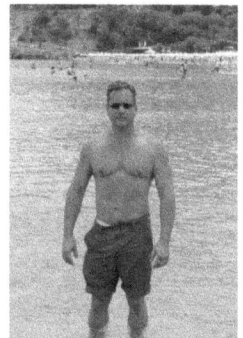
In Lindos, Greece at 57

Spartan Warrior Mindset

As an Ageless Warrior, I believe in the Spartan Warrior's way of not just being a strong, but looking great. The ancient Spartans inhabited what we call Greece today. The Spartans trained for war, had great looking bodies, and developed their minds. I believe that I'm a student for life. I'm on a never-ending quest to learn more about the martial arts, fitness, health, nutrition, weapons, and life. Just like Spartan Warriors that ate healthy, were intellectuals, trained for strength, maintained proportional bodies, trained with their weapons of war, and in hand-to-hand combat. I train with firearms, knife fighting, stand-up fighting, ground fighting, hand-to-hand combat, gun and knife defense, different fitness modalities, eat healthy, believe in developing the mind and train to have a body that looks good and looks strong.

I found a quote on Facebook by David Gemmell that summarizes the way I try to live my life and also summarizes what I wrote in the last paragraph about a Spartan Warrior's mindset. "A warrior...feeds his body well; he trains it; works on it. Where he lacks knowledge, he studies, but above all he must believe. He must believe in his strength of will, of purpose, of heart and of soul." Gemmell was a bestselling British author of heroic fantasy books.

Spartans lived fit and fearless. They believed in having a strong and well-proportioned, beautiful body. They glorified muscularity. This mindset is like bodybuilding. No, I don't mean today's competitive bodybuilders that weigh 250 to 300 pounds with two percent body fat. I feel that the Spartan mindset is more like the person that eats healthy and goes to the gym to develop more muscles in the right places to achieve a symmetrical yet strong body. I feel that even though the Spartans did not have bodybuilding competitions, they were the forefathers of bodybuilding due to their concept of a proportion muscular body and the statues that they built.The History of Sparta is from 950-192 B.C. To the Spartans, the development of the body was equally as important as development of the mind. The Spartans believed in "Sound Mind, Sound Body." They believed that being physically fit led to mental well-being, with the need for a strong, healthy body to have a sound mind.

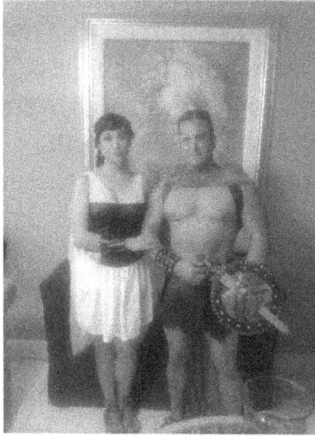

Going to costume party as Spartans
2012 Elena 42 and Julio 55 years old

Spartan boys and girls began special fitness programs by the age of six. The boys trained to strengthen their military skills and the girls trained for procreation. Spartans believed that knowledge, intellect and physical exercise was of equal value.

Spartans were one of the most physically fit soldiers in the history of world. The fitness goal of Sparta was not to produce athletes or soldiers. Their true goal was to produce men who were graceful, fit, and attractive. Their goal was to develop man that were fit for life.

The Spartans were courageous and had great strength. Three hundred Spartan warriors and their leader, King Leonidas, stopped King Xerxes and a million Persians. They fought to their death.

The Ageless Warrior fitness mindset is like being a Modern day Spartan. We must constantly develop and train the mind and body equally. We must have the determination to never give up even if the odds are against you. If you fail you must shake it off, get back up and continue to battle until you succeed. Remember this quote from the movie, *300*: "Madness? No, this is Sparta!" Some of your negative friends will not understand your dedication to become an Ageless Warrior. They will feel that you are going mad.

Workout for Longevity

When I first started bodybuilding, I admired the huge cut-up bodybuilders. I wanted to be like them, big and powerful – the bigger, the better. At my age, I'm not as impressed by a fit and ripped 20-something-year-old or a huge bodybuilder, even though I still admire them. In the years that I've been working out, I've seen the best athletes, most impressively built guys, and most beautiful and fit women become a shadow of themselves, unfit and overweight by the time they reach their 30's. Most of the great athletes and most popular kids in high school are unrecognizable by the time they reach their 40's. They are overweight and a shadow of what they were in high school.

I'm impressed and inspired by Jack LaLanne who was working out to stay fit right up until just a few days before his death. What impresses me is longevity – staying fit and healthy in your golden years. Health and fitness is not just for the young. As we get older, it's imperative to work out for longevity by warming up, staying away from injuries.

Working out for longevity doesn't mean working out with paper weight looking weights and kettlebells. If you saw the video of President Barack Obama at 52 years old working out in Poland you know what I mean. When we saw this on the national news, my wife argued with me that it wasn't the president, but instead, it was a comedian making fun of the president. Well, as we all know it was Obama working out with a chrome paperweight-like dumbbells. Most people believe that, that's the way you have to work out when you are in your 50's. I'm telling you that you do not have to train like Obama or join Planet Fitness when you are in your 50's even if you are the president.

Let's look at the opposite side of the spectrum. Vladimir Putin, the president of Russia, was born in October 2, 1952. Putin is a martial artist, participates in numerous sports, hunts, and also trains with heavy weights. He was the Leningrad Judo and Sambo champion. He is a six degree black belt in Judo, six degree black belt in Kyokushin Karate and is a Masters of Sport in Sambo. He has written a book on Judo and has no shame going shirtless in public.

I believe that if you work out like a 40-year-old or a 50-year-old you will look and feel like if you are 40 or 50. At 57, I look at the average 40 year old as an old man or woman and they look old to me. I don't place any limits on my training. Bruce Lee said, "If you always put limits on everything you do, physical or anything else, it will spread into your work and into your life. There are no limits. There are only plateaus, and you must not stay there, you must go beyond them."

Yet, in the last three years I've had to stop most of my functional training such as kettlebells, sledge hammer, tire flips, and others. As I've gotten older, I have had to adapt, improvise and overcome due to my injuries. My strength training is a modified bodybuilding workout. For cardio, I have a boxing coach. I train in Gracie Jiu Jitsu, and at my center, I teach kung fu, Muay Thai, Jeet Kune Do and Krav Maga. Throughout my life ever since I can remember, I've always had back pain. Yet, I've built my body around my back pain and other injuries.

As we age, we must be very careful how we train, who we train with, and where we train. Some martial arts and fitness programs can get you hurt, and as we age, it takes longer to recuperate from injuries. In my Krav Maga class, I have a 72-year-old man and a 68-year-old woman with double hip replacement and I make sure that they do not get injured.

How to Choose a Trainer or Fitness Program

I believe in leading by example. When choosing a fitness trainer the trainer should look the part. If you are looking for strength training, then the trainer should be strong. A martial arts instructor must also look fit and be able to demonstrate his techniques and they must be certified in their chosen field.

Be careful of young trainers that have never trained older clients. They need to understand longevity for that is how to truly train someone without injuring them. They need to know how to train you around your injuries. They need to know how to motivate and push you, yet not to the point of injury. It is better to find a trainer over 40 that leads by example, stays fit, and one who can relate to your body and injuries.

Today, many personal trainers are training clients in gyms, boxes, and martial arts studios using kettlebells and they have no idea what they are doing. I am amazed to see them use kettlebells like dumbbells. The positive part is that even though the kettlebell is not a dumbbell, they will most likely not get injured. My biggest problem is seeing those clueless trainers doing the staple of kettlebell training the swing totally wrong. Kettlebell training by a non-certified instructor is very dangerous and will cause injuries. We also have the Crossfit instructors with no kettlebell experience doing the craziest most dangerous moves. Most Crossfit instructors go to a weekend certification program and they start doing the WOD (workout of the day). If the WOD has kettlebells, they will do it, even though they don't have any experience training with kettlebells. There are exceptions like my good friend, Frank Demio, who has been certified in kettlebells since 2004 and owns Crossfit Gulf Coast The Cave in Sarasota, Florida, since 2005. Frank is an expert kettlebell trainer. The first kettlebell instructor training in Florida was done at my martial arts, fitness training center by kettlebell concepts. Frank and I were two of four people who were in this class.

Before starting to train in any fitness center or with a personal trainer, ask them if they have photos of the people they have trained. Do they have before and after photos of their clients? Are those photos of real people or just models? Stay away from franchises and affiliates. Be careful of franchises which sell the company or trainer a program, and use before and after photos that they bought or that were trained by the originator and not by them. This doesn't mean that they can get you in the shape of the models in their photos.

I was recently at a martial arts business seminar and an overweight, potbellied man who developed a fitness kickboxing affiliate program was trying to sell us an affiliation to his system. He claimed that he had 20 schools affiliated within his system. He had a few before and after photos, yet my question was: what happen to him? How could he try to sell us a kickboxing affiliation when he was not in shape? He was also bragging about how this was real kickboxing. The fit girl he was using in his video ad may have had good karate or tae kwon do kicks, but her boxing needed some serious work! If this is the person that the organization was showcasing, I'm sure the quality of their instructors nationally would even be worse.

I recommend instructors certified in Action Strength, MMA Fighter Fit, and Elite Combat Fitness which I'm certified in and know the instructors personally. The fitness program that I developed and is being taught in my martial arts and fitness center XFT (Xtreme Functional Training) MMA Fitness Boot Camp is a combination of the above mentioned programs with kickboxing, kettlebells, battling ropes and Indian clubs.

Avoid Negative People for Health and Success

For you to succeed in becoming an Ageless Warrior in life, you must avoid and stay away from negative people. We all have met them; we might even have family members like that. You know the ones that criticize all successful people. They feel that they have had bad luck in life. They say that they are better or more talented than the ones that have succeeded. They claim that they have not had the right breaks in life. The same way that they continue to talk about other people, they will eventually talk about you. They accuse the successful business people as being money hungry and living for the almighty dollar.

These are the same people who as soon as they know you are trying to succeed, change your lifestyle, or take up healthy activities, they will do their best to try to discourage you and tell you that you are too old. Never accept anything from anyone that you can't or shouldn't do it because of your age. Don't accept or listen to their negativity.

When I was training in kung fu in my mid-thirties I had friends tell me that I was too old to be doing kung fu. I had a co-worker tell me that I should get a part-time job instead of practicing kung fu. Some tried to make me feel guilty for training in kung fu. Little did they know that I had a vision and becoming a martial arts instructor was part of it. Today, due to following my instincts (and no listening to their negativity), I am more successful, financially stable and loving my career as a martial arts professional. The best thing that you can do is try to avoid those negative people while you are making the healthy lifestyle changes from this book.

Start building new relationships with other positive and successful people who will support, motivate and encourage you to succeed. I use to say that my wife and I got along well and had many friends that were difficult and negative. We tried to pray for them and help them. Yet, it always backfired and we ended up losing the relationship in a negative way. Since then, we have made it a point to be careful and stay away from those negative people. I strongly believe in this saying that I try to live by: "I will soar with the eagles and never again roll with the swine."

One of my favorite motivational speakers is Anthony Robbins. In one of his DVD's Robbins explained how, when he was poor, no one helped him when he had very little to eat. Now that he is successful and doesn't need it he rarely pays for a meal. People take him out for dinner and even when he's out eating on his own someone that has read his books or listened to his CD's ends up paying for his meals.

Let me tell you of a conversation that I had with Mike Mahler when I was driving him back to his hotel after a kettlebell seminar that he did at my martial arts fitness center. Mike is a world-renowned authority in kettlebell training, a strength coach, and also one of the nicest and most humble human beings that you can meet. He was talking to me about staying away from negative people and how he has had people criticize him for following his dreams and moving to California. They thought that he was crazy leaving a well-paying corporate job. He also shared with me that there are other people that claim that he is not qualified or schooled to be a strength coach or kettlebell instructor. He explained to me how being criticized is a sign that you are succeeding.

You must realize that you cannot succeed without others criticizing you. Anyone who is achieving a high level of success will be attacked, often viciously, and often for no reason other than the fact that the criticizer hates those who succeed. Those who invest time in criticizing others will never improve their own lives. Stay away from those people and don't let it bother you.

A few years ago I became friends on Facebook with a local Jeet Kune Do (JKD) instructor. Since my JKD instructor is in California I was thinking of also training with a local JKD instructor to take my JKD to another level. I was forewarned by a friend and JKD training partner about this negative instructor. The guy looked strong since he worked out with weights, yet was overweight. When I meet him he told me that he only had 8 JKD students. That should have been my wake up call. After a while, he started sending me texts telling me how great I could be if I had been training with him. One day I posted a JKD two-man flow drill that I learn from my first JKD instructor Paul Vunak who is one of the best and most recognize JKD instructors in the world. Paul has been called by Black Belt magazine, one of the best street fighters in the world and has been on the cover of Black Belt and other magazines. Vunak has trained numerous military and law enforcement agencies including Navy SEAL Team 6 in the 1980's. This negative instructor posted on my Facebook "Very nice, athletic, and acrobatic demo, but that's not Jeet Kune Do." I deleted the comment. Last year he texted me about doing a training section at my school since, he did not have a school any more. His idea was to do a workshop. He would teach JKD and I would teach Krav Maga. Since I did not answer him right away, he texted me the next day sarcastically saying, "Thanks for your answer." He was asking me to do a workshop at my school, but he gives me an attitude. I chose to ignore him. At New Years, he wrote me wishing me a happy New Year and asking me to do a workshop at my school. My assistant Krav Maga instructor put up a video of me doing a Krav Maga defense against a straight punch on Facebook. I had numerous martial arts and Krav Maga instructors give me positive comments and likes on this video. Once again, the negative instructor wrote to me: "That does not work in the street." Again, I deleted the message, but this time I finally de-friended him from my Facebook. I should have done this a few years ago. I'm sure this guy has low self-esteem and is envious of my success in the martial arts. Very few people outside of Miami know who he is.

One of the greatest things that has happened to me was separating from my first kung fu instructor. He was a very negative person. He was a master and one of the oldest students under our grand master's kung fu system, yet he was thrown out of the system after almost forty years under our grand master. I stayed loyal to our grand master until his death. I never called my former teacher and lost track of him. He later made up stories of our separation.

This kung fu instructor would curse his students out in class. He always hung out and was attracted other negative people. I remember one time, talking to a student who used the old cliché, "My Grandmother does better kung fu than that." Yet, he ended it with, "I'm not kidding she really does."

He would always tell me how terrible my kung fu was. When testing I would get nervous and make the silliest mistakes. I never won first place in a tournament when he was present. I had to go and compete on my own to be able to win first place trophies. I remember bringing him my first place trophy one day and he looked at my son who was 5 or 6 years old and told him, "Train hard so you will not be as bad as your father." I still regret how much he would intimidate me. I wish I could go back in time and change that.

He always bad-mouthed other martial artists and martial arts styles. In his mind, he was the greatest fighter ever and his system of kung fu was superior to all other martial arts. Most of his students believed that he was the greatest. For years, even I had been brainwashed to believe that he was the best. He did not want his students to weight train, because he said it would make them muscle-bound and slow. This was in the early nineties when most athletes were already training with weights.

He would tell us that no one could live off of teaching martial arts. I don't think that he ever had over 50 students at a time. He was very inconsistent. When I met him in the mid-1970's he had closed a school in New Jersey in order to move to Miami. His school in Hialeah, a neighboring city of Miami, lasted about a year and a half because he moved back to New Jersey. Even though after he left us, I studied different martial arts, I always remembered him and spoke to people about this extraordinary fighter. Around 16 years later in the early 1990's, I bumped into him at a Shaolin monk kung fu demonstration. Just like in the old chopsocky kung fu movies, I begged him to start teaching again. I started training at his house and within around 6 months he opened a storefront school. I put together the entire school for him, and with the help of my brother, Peter, and another old friend, and also a student from the 1970's, Jorge Cairo. That kung fu school stayed open for four and a half years.

His disciples (inner-circle students), which at one point might have been close to twenty-five, would have to cut his grass, do errands for him, and run to school for him. Sometimes he would spend weeks without showing up at the kung fu school. After the school closed, we would occasionally train with him, but he would show up one to two hours late. If you left before he got there he would get very upset. He even threw some people out of the system for not waiting for him or questioning him for being late.

He told us that he had met Bruce Lee twice at our Grand Master's teacher school in the 1960's in New York at the time that Bruce Lee was starring in *The Green Hornet*. He did not like Bruce Lee and claimed that Bruce Lee was a terrible martial artist. He said that when he was about 16 or 17 years old, he had an opportunity to speak with Bruce Lee. He said that he asked Lee why he left his foot out when kicking. Bruce looked at him up and down and said, "Movies, just movies." and walked away. He said that Bruce Lee was a jerk. I'm sure that what Lee meant with that remark was that he held his foot out for the effects on the TV screen. If Lee would have kicked and chambered the kick back in with his speed, the camera would have missed the details. I can only imagine what Bruce Lee must have thought, "Who the hell was this kid with a rude New Jersey accent? And to think he is questioning my kicking ability!"

This instructor was so close-minded that in the early 1990's when bottled water started to become popular, he would laugh and say how stupid Americans were and how smart the French were because the French were bottling water and charging for it and Americans are buying it when they could get it almost free from the sink. He would also argue that eating pork, lard and pork products was not un-healthy since in Cuba the country people in the farms would eat pork daily and live long, healthy lives. While I was still under him he had heart problems which lead to the need for a pace maker. Later, he was also diagnosed with Parkinson's disease.

As my school grew to about 300 students and I started to appear in numerous newspapers, magazines and TV shows I still never heard a praise or compliment from him. I thank God that I finally separated from this instructor and his semi-cultish school.
There is an old Spanish saying – let me try to translate it, "Tell me who you hang out with, and I'll tell you who you are." I also heard a motivational speaker say, "You will become the sum of the ten people you hang out with." This is so true. Eliminate negative people from your life and you will start attracting success!

Success Attracts Success

I remember many years ago, before I ran a successful martial arts and fitness center, I was having negative feelings and maybe a little bit of jealousy towards a person that I had just met. Here's how the story goes:

A good friend of my brother, whom I met when he was in his early teens, was inspired to work out with my brother and me when I was a competitive bodybuilder. Around 10 years ago, we were all at a party. He introduced his girlfriend to us. She had a master's degree from an ivy league school, had a successful business, was very successful, and was quite wealthy. Shortly after she started working out at a gym, a very well-known professional bodybuilding world champion that charged a high fee to train clients, started training her for free.

I told my wife that it was not fair for such a rich girl that could afford to pay a top bodybuilder for personal training to get it for free. I felt that she was so lucky to come out on the cover of a fitness magazine in the short time that she had been working out. I also went out to say that with all the years I had been bodybuilding, I was never on the cover of a magazine. In no time she became a fitness model and was on the cover of a bodybuilding magazine. I felt that she was so lucky. I also felt that it was unfair, since she could afford a trainer. Why would this top pro bodybuilder train her for free?

My wife's answer was that success attracts success. Later in life, I also learned that you become the sum of the ten people you hang out with. Today, I am very careful who I let into my inner circle. Since then, I've been on four magazine covers, one martial arts magazine, two fitness magazines, a local magazine, front pages of numerous newspapers, and I've been on over 150 TV shows. Believe me success attracts success. What my wife, Elena, meant was that successful people attract other successful people.

Protect your Inner Circle for Success

You become the sum of the ten people you hang out with, so it is of vital importance to protect your inner circle. Your inner circle are your friends and family members that you are closest to. We've already talked about staying away from negative people and how success attracts success.

Let me continue with another Anthony Robbins story. In a DVD series I heard Robbins talk about the time when a General, the commanding officer of Camp Lejeune, called him to talk to the Marines. Robbins was humbled, yet amazed. He felt that he did not know what to say to the greatest fighting men in the world. They are already highly dedicated and truly motivated. The General told him that when they were in the Marine Corps they held higher standards since they were around likeminded, high-achieving motivated peers. The problem was that after they got discharged and were no longer keeping company with high-achieving peers, their standards quickly dropped and most of them did not continue to achieve their goals.

That is why you must protect your inner-circle. I have some very successful people that I have allowed to enter my inner circle. Let me tell you about a few of my inner-circle, close friends.

My pastor and spiritual leader is Bobby Cruz, Jr.. Bobby is not just a close and great friend, but he is also my spiritual mentor. I met my wife, Elena, in church. One year later, while still dating Elena, my sister Marietta Slentz Anta started attending a church called *Iglesia Casa de Alabanza* which was pastored by Bobby Cruz and Richie Ray. Before becoming Christians, Bobby and Richie were the top Salsa performers. My wife and I were baptized and married by Richie. Four years later, we left to join another church. In the next seventeen years attended two other churches. Finally, we came back to *Casa de Alabanza*. The new pastor was Bobby Cruz's son, Bobby Jr..

Bobby Jr. was also our next-door neighbor. Within a short time we became close friends. Bobby Jr. and I have a lot in common. Bobby Jr. is 50 yet looks younger and stays in shape by lifting weights and jogging.

Bobby Jr. has given me great spiritual, marital, and parenting tips. I'll never forget one time that I had a problem and was very upset and stressed out. My wife was very concerned for me. As I was driving, I received a call from Bobby Jr... He said, "Hey, Julio! I was just calling to see how you are doing." I had to laugh and I asked him if my wife had called him about my situation. Right after my wife had called him, he called me to give me advice, comfort and to pray for me. I have never had a pastor do that before. Yet, he is not just a pastor, but a close friend and part of my inner circle.

Alfred Magnon is a 6'4" gentle giant, close friend and part of my inner circle. He is my martial arts training partner. In 2007, seven year before the writing of this book, I received a call from Alfred. He told me that he was a martial artist that he was planning to open a school in a few years. He wanted to meet with me since at that time I was NAPMA's (National Association of Professional Martial Artist) NSSN Florida state representative. Alfred helped me by judging at my inner school tournament. I helped him and mentored him in his martial arts business. When I first met Alfred, he was a black belt in Kenpo Karate, a blue belt in Gracie Jiu Jitsu, and had trained in Jeet Kune Do and Muay Thai Kickboxing. I held the rank of Kung Fu Master and was a certified Haganah Israeli Self Defense instructor. I believed in cross training and had played around with boxing, kickboxing and a little Brazilian Jiu Jitsu. I had an interest in Jeet Kune Do and Muay Thai. Through Alfred's influence we both became interested in getting certified in Muay Thai. I went to train at the MAIA Super Show in Las Vegas with Master Toddy and Alfred went to his Muay Thai certification. I decided to get certified with Master Tran. Around four years later in 2013 Alfred and I both got certified as Kru's Level 3 Muay Thai instructors under the Tran Muay

Thai Kickboxing Association. Alfred's guidance and motivation were important factors to get both of us involved and certified in Paul Vunak's Jeet Kune Do. Later, we both trained under the Jeet Kune Do Athletic Association. I also started training with Alfred in Gracie Jiu Jitsu at Valenti Brothers Jiu Jitsu.

I rarely let a student become part of my inner circle because it usually doesn't turn out well. With Mike Catala and his family I made an exception. Mike came to my school in his mid-forties. He was a successful salesman for Bristol Myers, yet he was overweight and out of shape. Mike started in my Muay Thai program and now he does Muay Thai and Krav Maga. He also motivated his family to start training his wife and two of his three sons are training in our program. Mike is now fit and fearless and is a close likeminded friend. Mike is teaching me and advising me on how to invest in the stock market.

One day I received a call from my friend, strongman and power lifting champion, Bud Jeffries. Bud tells me that he has a friend, Eric Guttman, who is a naval officer that has orders to go to Miami. He told me that he will be stationed in South Cam (Southern Command). Southern Command is located in the same city in which I live, Doral. When I met Eric, he told me that Daryl and Kim Brown and Bud Jeffries had told him that when he arrived in Miami, he had to make time to meet me. Kim and I trained together at Moni Aizik's Elite Combat Fitness certification.

Eric and I have become close friends. We share martial arts, fitness, anti-aging, health, and nutrition information. Since Eric has authored two books and an instructional video he has inspired me to start writing this book.

Unfortunately I have had to push some people out of my inner circle and had to do so with a very heavy heart. I would talk to them if I bump into them somewhere, but I would love them from a distance.

Chapter 2
Getting Fit and Fearless

Don't you realize that your body is the temple of the Holy Spirit, who lives in you and was given to you by God? You do not belong to yourself.

1 Corinthians 6:19

Optimal Fitness for an Ageless Body

For optimal fitness, an Ageless Warrior must train to obtain strength, cardiovascular endurance, joint mobility, flexibility and balance. 80% of your success will be obtained by healthy eating. Stay away from cigarettes, alcohol and drugs. I don't smoke or do drugs and rarely drink alcohol. I was never an alcoholic. In my twenties, before I became a Christian, I would drink at clubs. After I became a Christian, I didn't have a drink for around 20 years. After reading about how wine can be beneficial to your health and help you relax, I felt that a little red wine once in a blue moon wouldn't hurt. I might drink a glass of wine every two or three months. For optimal health, try to closely follow my Ten Commandments of Health and Fitness which I will describe later on in this chapter.

"Exercise is king, nutrition is queen and together you've got a kingdom." – Jack LaLanne.

The purpose of writing this book is to inspire you and lead you on your quest for longevity, health and an ageless body. As a student for life I have dedicated my life to health, fitness and personal defense. To obtain optimal fitness wouldn't be easy especially if you have an assortment of medical conditions which could be aggravated by exercise. I have pain in my neck, shoulder, back and thumb. I live in pain. Whether I exercise or not, I'm still going to have pain. So, I chose to exercise. I just train around my injuries.

As you advance in age, more problems become prevalent due to poor lifestyle choices or injuries. You must stay active and train around your injuries. Staying active, exercise and nutrition is the Fountain of Youth. Nothing does more for our quality of life and longevity than staying active as we age. Your mindset is of optimal importance. If you think like an old person, you'll feel old and train like an old person. So, you'll act and look old.

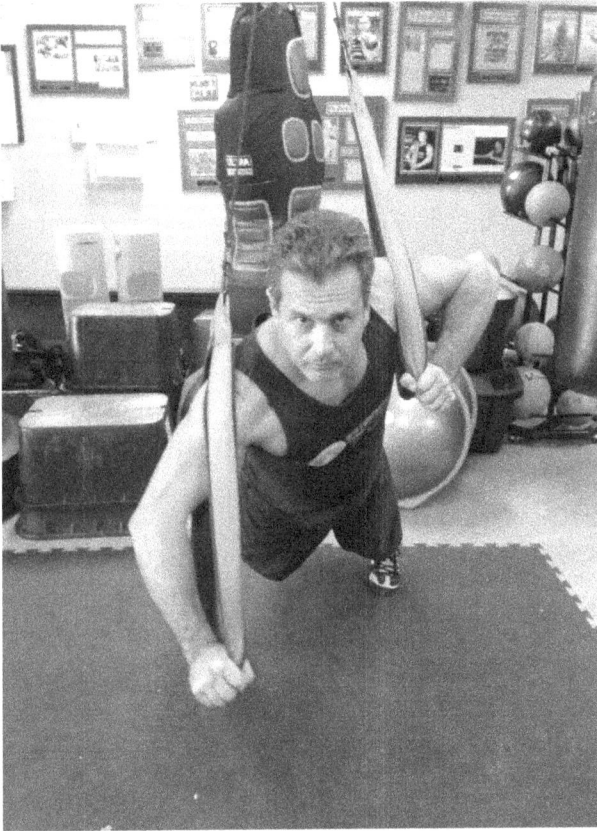

The key to staying young and fit is persistency. Start slow and take it one step at a time. We've had people come to our exercise classes and overdo it the first day and never come back. I've notice that at times people that start super excited and

Airfit Training in 2013

motivated slowly give up and sizzle away. Confucius said, "It doesn't matter how slow you go as long as you do not quit." Remember that the rabbit was fast, but he came in last after the turtle. Consistency is the key to success.

Get Motivated

The only way to succeed is by making a lifestyle change. In the beginning you will need some self-discipline to start eating healthy and exercising on a regular basis. With time discipline becomes a habit and a lifestyle.

When I was a small boy I remember hating to brush my teeth, but I also remember my parents reprimanding me and trying to explain to me the importance of hygiene. Today it's part of my routine to wake up and brush my teeth. I cannot see myself leaving my house without brushing my teeth. In the same way, I cannot see myself not doing my strength training and martial arts training five to six days a week. Habits we train are habits we obtain.

Your success will come if you want it bad enough. You have to make a decision today to change your lifestyle. If you were to stand nude in a full length mirror right now, would you be happy with what you are looking at? I know this sounds weird and freaky, but be honest with yourself. Do you like what you see?

Standing naked in front of a mirror is one of two mental exercises you must do to motivate yourself to change and make working out and healthy eating a lifestyle. So, if you haven't done it yet, get naked, analyze your body and get ready to change what you see. Visualize the body that you want to have. (Oh, and by the way, please make sure you are at home in your room or bathroom before you take your close off. I sure would not want you writing me about how you were arrested for indecent exposure!)

The second drill I want you do, is to close your eyes and visualize. Your mind is your most powerful muscle. Every great thing, discovery, or invention had its beginning in someone's mind. With your eyes closed visualize, how you will look and feel in a month, three months, six months and a year if you follow the Ageless Warrior fitness lifestyle. Now, with your eyes closed, visualize how you will look and feel after one month, three months, six months and even a whole year if you simply continue to live your life doing what you been doing for all these years. Think how heavy you will become and how unhealthy you will be.

You must always have positive thoughts. The Bible says, "As a man thinketh in his heart, so is he" (Proverb 23:7 KJV). It is important to watch your words. The Bible also states, "But those things which proceed out of the mouth come forth from the heart; and they defile the man" (Matthew 15:18 NIV)

I suggest that you listen to motivational speakers in order to stay positive and motivated through life. I listen to motivational CD's in my car as I drive. My favorite motivational speakers are Anthony Robbins and Zig Ziggler.

Let me quote the king of kung fu, Bruce Lee, "If you spend too much time thinking about a thing, you'll never get it done." Here are some great quotes:

"Vision without execution is just hallucination." Henry Ford.
"Stay motivated, believe and expect change in your body and life." Zig Ziggler
"Motivation is like bathing, you must do it every day or it will wear off." Zig Ziggler
"If you do what you've always done, you'll get what you've always gotten." Tony Robbins

Now, just stop thinking about it and stop having doubts. Let's set a date for action, by starting a date to exercise, joining a martial arts school that specializes in fitness, and by starting a healthy eating plan now. Write up a contract with yourself concerning your commitment to change your lifestyle by eating healthy foods and exercising, and then sign that contract.

Anta's Ten Commandments of Health and Fitness

1. **Faith/Vision**

2. **Healthy Life Style Peaceful Living/Rest**

3. **Eat Healthy Foods**

4. **Water**

5. **Functional Anaerobic Exercising**

6. **Aerobic Exercising**

7. **Stretching/Joint Mobility**

8. **Breathing Exercise**

9. **Sunshine**

10. **Fasting**

To acquire optimal fitness you must have low body fat, muscular endurance, muscular strength, joint mobility, balance, and flexibility. This in return will keep you strong, healthy, and free from disease and injury to live a longer and more abundant life. I've been involved in fitness and martial arts for over 40 years. I'm the first to admit that I have made lots of mistakes, yet through those mistakes I have learned to succeed. Below is an explanation of each my ten Commandments of Health and Fitness. Follow these ten guidelines lines to acquire optimum fitness.

1. Faith/Vision
You must believe and have faith that you will succeed. The more you fail and the more you are rejected, the closer you are

to victory. Vision is a dream or goal with a deadline. Write your vision with your goals and never lose sight of them.

The Bible says, "And the Lord said to me, Write my answer on a billboard, large and clear, so that anyone can read it at a glance and rush to tell the others. But these things I plan won't happen right away. Slowly, steadily, surely, the time approaches when the vision will be fulfilled. If it seems slow, do not despair, for these things will surely come to pass. Just be patient! They will not be overdue a single day!" (Habakkuk 2:2-3, The Living Bible)

I been writing my vision ever since 1996. One day while working as a Corrections Officer at South Florida Reception Center, a fellow officer and good friend, Eric Gonzales, came to me all excited to share the message on vision from Habakkuk 2:2-3 which his pastor had given in church. That was the day that changed my life. Since I started writing my vision and having faith, my life changed. I have continued to write my vision every December since the day Eric brought that Bible verse to me.

2. Healthy Life Style
Your body is your temple. If you don't take care of your body where would you live?

No Vice Stay away from drinking alcohol, smoking or drug use. Eliminate soft drinks.

Peaceful Living Find a private place to have a peaceful time for yourself to relax and pray. Eat in a peaceful environment with good company. Eat slowly and chew your food twenty to fifty times. I must confess I am guilty of not chewing my food enough. This is a bad habit I got in Marine Corps boot camp where they gave us little time to eat. Sometimes I'm guilty of chewing my foot 3 or 4 times before swallowing. But, I'm working on it.

Rest Work and play hard six days a week but make sure you take one day off for rest and relaxation. Even the almighty God rested on the seventh day. Get a good night's sleep every day. The body repairs while you sleep.

No Negative Thoughts or People Think positive. Keep all negative thoughts, such as fear, hate and envy, out of your mind. FEAR is False Expectations Appearing Real. Negative people will keep you from success. Keep them away from you and your life.

3. Eat Healthy Foods

We all know what healthy foods and unhealthy foods are. Foods as close to the way God made them are healthy. Man-made, processed, refined and altered foods are unhealthy. Eat organic as much as possible.

4. Water

Drink at least eight to ten glasses of pure water every day. Our bodies are almost 85% water. Next to oxygen, water is the most important element for staying alive. We can't survive without it.

5. Functional Anaerobic Exercising

Functional training is the way that we use our bodies daily by using different muscles simultaneously. Examples of some functional exercises are kettlebells, Olympic Weight Lifting, Pilates, Indian Club Swinging, Rope Climbing and Calisthenics. Muscle specific weight machine training is not functional, yet it is a lot better than sitting around the house eating and channel surfing. If you have injuries like me, then this will be what keeps you fit.

6. Aerobic Exercising

You need no more than twenty minutes of aerobic workout per day to stay in good cardiovascular shape. Sprinting, kettlebell training, swimming and riding a bicycle will give you an aerobic workout. Keep your cardio workouts fun and functional. To make sure that you get speed, bursting power and balance in your workout, so stay away from fixed bicycles and treadmills unless you do interval training on them.

7. Stretching/Joint Mobility
Stretching relaxes your body, reduces muscle tension, increase range of motion, prevents injury, promotes circulation and reduces lactic acid that is produced after a workout. Great forms of stretching are Kung Fu, Tai Chi, Pilates and Yoga. Stretching is the most neglected physical activity.

8. Breathing Exercise
Oxygen is the most important element keeping us alive. You cannot survive more than a few minutes without oxygen. Go outdoors and breathe fresh air daily. Pilates, Yoga, Tai Chi, kung fu and Chi Gong will teach you great techniques for healthy breathing.

9. Sunshine
The sun is a powerful healer. It kills germs and relaxes you. It helps your body absorb calcium and it creates vitamin D. Remember that light brings life and darkness brings death. I love sunbathing at the beach and even in back yard.

10. Fasting
Fasting is a physical and spiritual cleansing process. Fasting gives your digestive track a break. This is one of my weaknesses that I'm working on.

Strength Training

Warriors have been strength training for thousands of years. Ancient Greek and Roman soldiers would lift rock to strengthen their bodies. Milo of Croton, a Greek wrestler, in the sixth century began lifting a calf. As the calf grew, Milo became stronger. By the time that the calf became a cow, Milo had become much stronger and was able to lift the cow. It is said that this was the beginning of progressive strength training. The Shaolin monks of China trained with heavy padlocks.

Strength training can be done with weights, kettlebells, sandbags, or body weight training Strength training will help you strengthen your bones and maintain and build muscle. Heavy weight training will help you raise your testosterone levels. To increase your testosterone levels through weight training you'll want to increase the weight and lower your number of reps.

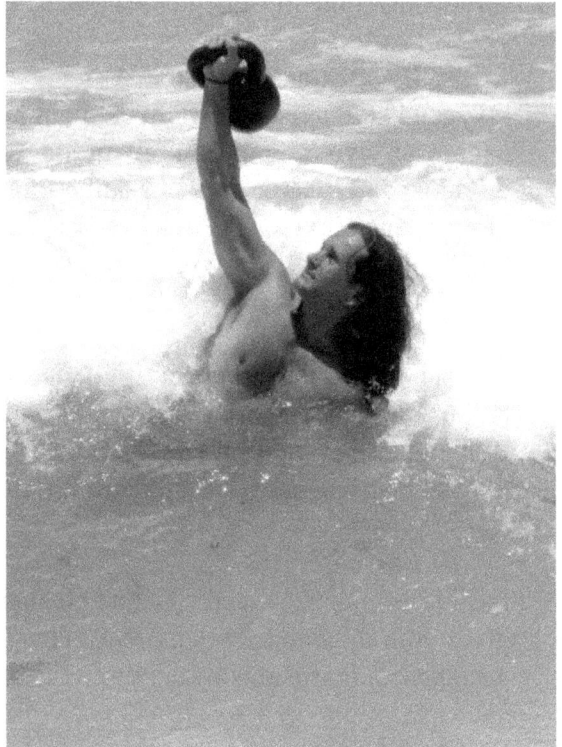

Focus on compound moves that work a wider number of muscles, such as squats, clean and press and dead lifts with barbells or kettlebell movements. If you have injuries like I do, you might not be able to do those lifts. Even though I'm not naturally strong and cannot do squats, dead lifts or clean and press, I still train heavy with low repetitions.

One of the great benefits of strength training is muscle building. There have been numerous studies on how larger muscles burn calories. One study said that for every pound of muscle you have, you will burn 50 calories in a day. Another study said that one pound of muscle burns about 6.5 calories per hour. The truth of the matter is that muscle burns more calories than fat. Building muscle is extremely important in burning fat.

The larger the muscles the more you can eat. Having large muscles speeds up your metabolism. When your metabolism is faster you will lose weight faster and you'll also be able to eat more.

When my younger brother, Peter, and I went to Columbus, Ohio for UFC 82 and The Arnold Sports Festival on March 1, 2008, we had the opportunity to meet Jay Cutler, bodybuilding champion and four-time Mr. Olympia. "Mr. Olympia" is the title for the most prestigious professional bodybuilding event. A friend of my brother is one of Jay's closest friends. Jay's friend is also a friend of my brother's business partner, Jeff Johnson, who is from Columbus, Ohio. My brother called Jeff to tell him that their mutual friend from Miami was in Columbus. My brother and I went from the Arnold Sports Festival to The UFC. After the UFC, we called Jeff to pick us up. Jeff told us that he was at a restaurant with Cutler and their mutual friend. When we arrived, I was greatly impressed to see Jay eating his second large steak and potato plate. This plate could have been shared by any two adults and they would have been satisfied yet Cutler had two plates. If I were to eat that way, I would be obese; yet Jay has to eat that much to fuel his muscular body. Jay is 5'9" weighs 310 pounds in his off season, and 274 pounds in contest shape.

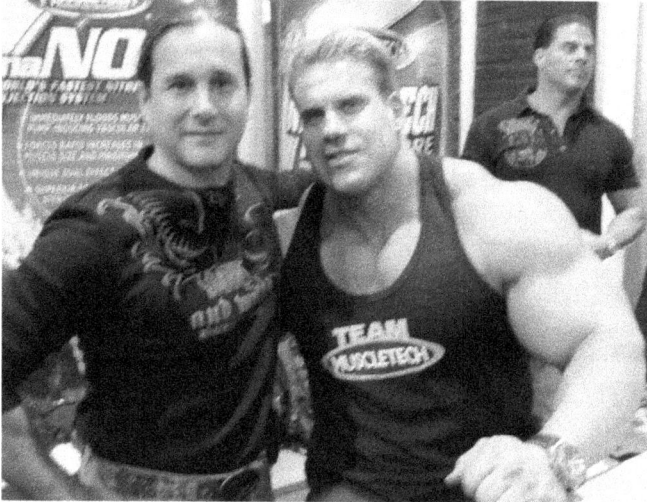

With Jay Cutler in 2008

In our 30's, we begin to lose muscle mass at around a one-half to one percent each year and it only worsens as we get into our late 50's and early 60's. This is known as sarcopenia. By the time we turn 60, we could lose around thirty percent of our muscle. This in turn will slow down your metabolism and cause you to gain weight and look soft and weak. By doing proper strength training you will significantly reduce the loss of muscle. If you train like an Ageless Warrior rather than training like a senior citizen, you can gain muscle as I have. Strength training will strengthen your bones, reduce your risks from arthritis and osteoporosis, and improve your balance, posture and coordination. I especially like the fringe benefit of looking muscular and good.

Strength training is ideal for the Ageless Warrior. It builds and retains muscle mass, strengthens your bones, increases your testosterone, increases HGH, and speeds up your metabolism.

Functional Training or Bodybuilding Type Workout

Those that train in functional training make fun of bodybuilders for being buff and muscular. They claim that bodybuilder's muscles are not functional. Bodybuilders laugh at those that do functional training saying that they have to write on social media what they accomplish in training because you cannot tell that they are strong by looking at their bodies, yet you can recognize a bodybuilder anywhere because of their great looking body and muscularity. Bodybuilding for seniors is now being called the "fountain of youth" since these seniors have bodies that look better and are actually more muscular than athletes in their twenties.

I agree with both those who advocate bodybuilding and those who advocate functional training. I was a competitive bodybuilder in the 1980's and certified as a personal trainer. I'm certified in numerous functional training modalities such as kettlebells, Indian clubs, Battling Ropes, Pilates, Fitness Kickboxing, Elite Combat Fitness, Action Strength and MMA Fighter Fit. The first kettlebell instructor trainer course in the state of Florida took place at my training center in June 2004, by Kettlebell Concepts. I have been certified in kettlebells by three different kettlebell organizations.

Both bodybuilders and function training enthusiasts have a good point. Why would anyone want to have a great looking muscular body, yet not be able to run up a flight of stairs? Why would anyone want to climb ropes, jump over walls, and run miles, yet look like a pencil neck geek? I personally want to be functionally fit and also look the part.

I have always told my martial arts students: "What is it worth to have the best built body in the world and then get killed by a thug because you do not know how to defend yourself? What is it worth to be the greatest fighter in the world, but die of a heart attack do to obesity?" The late great Bruce

Lee is an example of a man ahead of his time. When most martial artist and athletes were against weight training, Lee was cross training in various kinds of martial arts, doing a bodybuilder's workout, and practicing functional training. He did one arm pushups on one finger, and he performed the dragon fly and numerous other bodyweight functional movements.

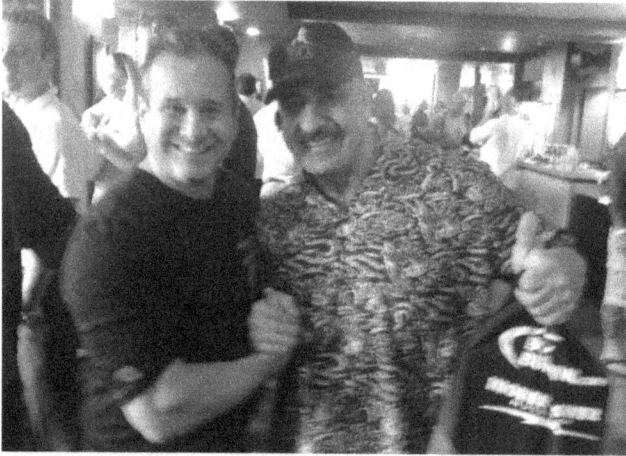

With Samir Bannout in 2012

In December 2012, I went to see the Masters Mr. Olympia. This is the highest level of competition for professional bodybuilders over the age of 40. While in the audience, I met many of the bodybuilders that I had admired while I was competing in the 1980's. The most charismatic bodybuilder I met was the 1983 Mr. Olympia, Samir Bannout who will be 59 at the end of this year. I was a huge fan of Samir. Samir is still in great shape after all these years. When I met him, I told him that the year in which he won the title of Mr. Olympia, I had competed in my first bodybuilding show and that I was 56 years old. My brother, Peter, jokingly said, "Yeah, my brother is quite an old man!" Samir responded by saying, "No, your brother looks great. Bodybuilding keeps him young." I fully agree with Samir. Bodybuilding does keep you young by building muscles.

The old-time bodybuilders did strongman feats, but they also performed acrobats. A perfect example is Eugene Sandow (April 2, 1867 – October 14, 1925). Sandow was a pioneer bodybuilder and has been referred to as the "father of modern bodybuilding." Even in the 1940's, there were bodybuilders doing acrobatics and feats of strength in Venice Beach, California, famously known as "Muscle Beach."

I believe in the best of both worlds. I believe that bodybuilding helps you builds the best body in the fastest way. I also believe that functional training under a trained certified instructor will keep you agile and moving functionally. If you combine bodybuilding with functional training, you'll look but you will also move and feel great.

My only concern about some functional training systems is the over-emphasis on competition and breaking your record and time during each workout. They perform high-repetition Olympic lifting when Olympic lifting was never intended for high repetition. They also do kettlebell training until exhaustion; yet first rule of kettlebell training is to stop before you become tired. Our goal is to train injury- free and to train for longevity.

Due to my back injury, I am training more like a bodybuilder today. I am still able to train and teach different martial arts such as Krav Maga, Muay Thai, Jeet Kune Do, Kung Fu and Gracie Jiu Jitsu; but I cannot do kettlebells, dead lifts or barbell squats. At 57 years old, I stay muscular by using other bodybuilding types of workouts.

I strongly believe in functional training, unless you have certain injuries. Regardless, of whatever injury you might have, you can still train around it with a modified bodybuilding type workout at home or at a gym.

Beginner's Bodybuilding Type Workout Routine

This routine is for a beginner that has never done strength training or for someone who has not worked out in over a year. To use this type of workout, you must be healthy and without any kind of injuries. (If you are injured or extremely out of shape, follow the alternate workout which I explain later in this chapter.) This beginner's bodybuilding type of workout will also work for the "hard gainer" – a person who has not yet been able to see any gains in their workout. Each body part needs at least forty-eight hours of rest to recuperate. This workout is a split routine. It can be done on Monday, Tuesday, Thursday and Friday. You will rest on Wednesday, Saturday and Sunday.

This routine was given to me by Mario Ramil who had 18 inch arms in high school. Mario called it "Prehistoric Training" He did this routine for years. He told me that it was given to him by a Spaniard. He did the entire routine with the exception of calves and abs three times a week, Mondays, Wednesdays, and Fridays in his backyard. I modified it and made it a push and pull split routine. You work half of the body on one day and work the other half of the body on the next day. On one day you will train the pulling muscles and the day following you will train the pushing muscles.

This split routine can be done at a home gym. All that is needed is a barbell and a bench. It could be modified if you have any injuries. You can also modify it by substituting dumbbells for some or even all of these exercises.

If you do not currently strength train, or you have not been strength training in a long while, or if you are not in good shape, then you should start with only three sets per exercise and add one set every week until you reach the six sets. If you are currently strength training, but you are not seeing results, then you can do the program as written. Do this program for 6 to 12 months.

Monday & Thursday			
Body Part	**Exercise**	**Sets**	**Reps**
Chest	Bench Press	6	6
Shoulders	Front Shoulder Press	6	6
Triceps	Close Grip Bench Press	6	6
Abdominals	Superset Leg Raises with Crunches	3	20

Tuesday & Friday			
Body Part	**Exercise**	**Sets**	**Reps**
Thighs	Squats	6	6
Calves	Calf Raises	6	6
Lats *(Upper Back)*	Bent over rows	6	6
Biceps	Curls	6	6

If you are totally out of shape, obese, or have injuries and cannot follow this workout, then here is an alternative bodyweight workout. This alternative workout is for someone that does not have the strength, health, or coordination to do the beginner's workout.

This alternate workout can be done in 10 to 20 minutes two to three times a week. Allow at least 48 hours between each day of workout. Two to three times a week on the days in which you do not do this alternate strength workout, walking would be a good exercise.

Depending on your fitness level start with one, two, or three sets of as many repetitions as you can do with good form.

Squat to chair: Put a chair behind you. Push your hips back as far as you can. Then bend your knees. When your glutes touch the chair, come back up to the starting position. Do not sit down on the chair. Use the chair as a reference point.

Pushups: If you can do regular pushups, do them. If you cannot do regular pushups, do modified pushups and build up to regular pushups. Here are some easier pushups in order of difficulty: Pushups with legs open, pushups on your knees and pushups standing against a wall.

Crunches: Most people can do crunches. Lay on your back with your hands crossed in front of your chest. Have your chin touch your chest. Exhale bring your scapula off the ground and squeeze your abdominals. Then return to the starting position on your back.

After you are comfortable with this workout, you can start the calisthenics bodyweight workout on page 81. After you are proficient with the calisthenics routine, you'll be ready for the beginner's bodybuilding workout. Longevity and safety are of the utmost importance in the Ageless Warrior Fitness workout. It is better to start slow and attain your goals, than to get injured and have to stop training.

My Current Bodybuilding Type Routine

My current workout is built around my injuries. If I had no injuries, it would be ideal to do barbell squats, barbell dead lifts and kettlebells to build muscle and bring up my testosterone level. When I train with kettle bells my strength increases and I don't have to do any cardio since a kettlebell workout is both aerobic and anaerobic. Due to my injuries, I've learned to adapt, improvise and overcome.

I train instinctively by changing my routine around. Sometimes I try to lift heavy and explosive, while on other occasions I'll go slow and resist in the negative part of the exercise. At times I superset. A superset is doing two separate exercises for the same body part without resting in between sets. I'll also go on a machine up and down the rack, to increase the weight without rest for a set or two. I do this if I'm in hurry or looking for a good pump.

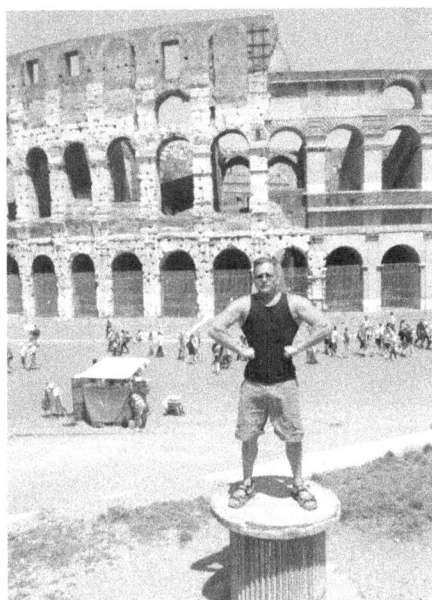

Striking a pose at the Colosseum in Rome 2014

My workout, depending on the body part on which I am focusing, takes between 30 and 45 minutes. I train each body part once a week. I used to train each body part twice a week in my competitive bodybuilding days. As I've gotten older, I feel that I need more rest for proper recuperation. I work out with weights five day a week from Monday through Friday. Today I'm more aware of my body and after over thirty years of not being able to bench press I am now benching today. Normally, bringing the bar down to touch the chest is the proper way to

69

bench press, but for my situation, how heavy I bench and whether I let the bar touch my chest or not depends on how my shoulders feel.

Below is a sample of a bodybuilding style workout that I'm currently doing:

Monday: Lats (upper back) 16 Sets

Pull-ups 3x failure

Front Lat Pull-down 1x12-15

Front Lat Pull-downs and Standing Front Lat Pull-downs Superset 3x6-8

Barbell Bent Over Rows 3X6

Seated Low Lat Pull to Stomach

I'll also do lower back and abs depending on how my back is feeling,

Tuesday: Legs

Quads (front of thigh) 22 Sets Total

Leg Extension 1x 12-20

Leg Extension 5x6-10

Leg Press Machine 5x6-8

Adductor Machine 3x6-8

Abductor Machine 3x6-8

Hamstrings (back of thigh)

Seated Leg Curls 5x6-10

Calves: It varies depending on where I train

Wednesday: Shoulders and Traps

Shoulders 16 Sets Total

To warmup, I do a light giant set of 4x 10-15, lateral raises, Arnold presses, bend over rows and front lateral raises.

Side Lateral Raises Super Set with Arnold Press with dumbbells 4x6-8

Side Lateral Front Lateral Raise Combo 3x6-8 (Start the move with side lateral raises and bring it down with front lateral raises)

Machine Rear Delt Flies 4x6-8

Traps 5 Sets Total

Shrugs 5x 6-8

Thursday: Biceps and Triceps

Biceps 16 Sets Total

Warmup light dumbbell curls or e-z curl bar curls 1x15

EZ-curl bar standing curls 4x6-8

Bicep Dumbbell Curls Superset with Hammer Curls 4x6-8

Preacher curl machine (Scott Curl) 3x6-8

Triceps 16 Sets Total

Tricep cable press-downs 1X15

Tricep cable press downs Superset with reverse cable press downs 4X6-8

Close Grip Bench Press 4X6-8

Seated Tricep Extension Machine 3X6-8

Friday: Chest

Barbell Bench Press 1X10-20

Barbell Bench Press 3X6-8

Incline Bench Press, barbell or dumbbell 5X6-8

Seated Flies machine 6X6-10

I gave this workout to my friend, Joe Chao, who is 51. Chao and I meet in college. We became good friends in 1993 training in the same kung fu school. We got our first black belts together in Hung Gar Kung Fu. We both started teaching kung fu and fitness kickboxing in 1998. I continued teaching and studying other martial arts, yet he stopped teaching due to his primary job. Two years ago, Joe started training at my school in Muay Thai and Krav Maga and started helping me in class.

After hearing my philosophy that a martial arts instructor must lead by example and look the part, he started to work out with weights seriously. Joe didn't feel that he was getting many results and asked me for a weight training routine. He told me that he trains hard, yet he never sees much muscular growth. He wrote down his routine and asked me what I thought about it. I looked at it and asked him to explain to me how he worked out, how long he would stay at the gym and how many sets and repetitions he does. After listening to him, I gave him a workout similar to the one that I'm currently doing. I had him train heavier and lower his repetitions. Two weeks after doing this routine he told me how much muscle growth he was noticing. He also wrote on Facebook "Second week using the five-day split routine that Julio Anta created for me. I have to tell you that even my wife has noticed some development. Thank you, Julio Anta."

Even as I am finishing the writing of this book, I am changing my workout. Due to my Brazilian Jiu Jitsu, boxing, Tai Chi, and the time it takes to run a successful martial arts fitness center, I am putting together a gym in my garage. This in turn will help me save time by not having to drive to the gym. I will also be able to work out any time I like. My workout will change according to the equipment that I have in my garage. I

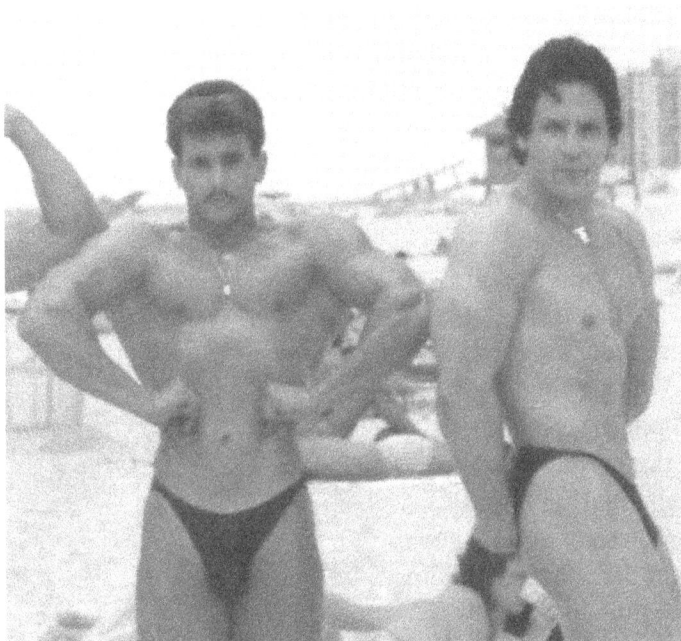

In 1983 with my training partner and trainer Smokee Joe Travie

promise to keep my readers posted on my training on my blog, "MartialArtsAndFitness.typepad.com" and on my Facebook fitness group, "Anta's Health, Strength and Fitness."

Kettlebells

Kettlebells (referred to as Girya in Russia, KB's, and also K-bells) are the ultimate training tool for the Ageless Warrior because they will help you build real world strength, speed, conditioning, endurance and work capacity. Regardless of whether you do martial arts as a traditional martial artist, or in quest of a UFC title or winning gold in the Olympics, or you are defending yourself in the streets, or perfecting your forms, kicking higher, faster and stronger. or if you are merely just trying to stay injury free, kettlebells are your perfect companion. Kettlebells are the perfect workout for the martial artist regardless of style, age or gender. They will help you build speed, power, cardiovascular fitness and flexibility to make you a better and stronger. Kettlebells have

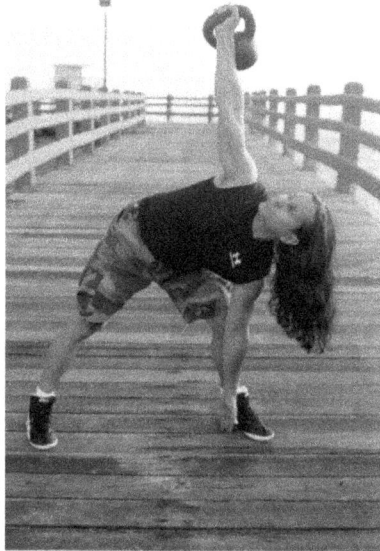

Kettlebell Training in South Beach 2006

been growing in popularity with athletes and the Hollywood elite. You might have seen them in scenes from the movies, "Rocky Balboa," and "Never Back Down," or possibly in the pre-fight clips of UFC fighters training.

My fascination with kettlebells began over 11 years ago. Being a former competitive bodybuilder, I believe that martial arts and fitness are one. I'm always looking for a great workout. When I was a young kid, my two loves were bodybuilding and martial arts. I first heard about kettlebells in the early 1970's, but I did not hear about it again until over thirty years later.. As a kid and teenager I would read all the muscle and karate magazines available in the 1970's. All the muscle magazines of the early 1970's sold barbell, dumbbell sets with kettlebell handles. I also remember seeing strongmen lifting kettlebells in vintage photos from the turn of the last century. In 2003, Kathy Mahler, a friend of mine from Clearwater, Florida, called me to assist her in a Women's self-defense seminar for a fitness conference in Miami. While at the conference, I participated in a kettlebell workshop and I was hooked. It was not until 2004 that I was able to begin training with kettlebells. That year, the first kettlebell instructor training in the state of Florida was held at my school by Kettlebell Concepts making me a kettlebell pioneer in South Florida. At that time, I started the first group kettlebell class and kettlebell website www.MiamiKettlebell.com in Miami.

Kettlebells are a unique power tool for everyone because they are usually not meant to be lifted like weights rather than to be swung. Life in general is full of movements, kettlebell workouts mimic life movements. They incorporate a human's six natural movements which are squat, push, lunge, pull, bend and twist. kettlebells are unlike the two dimensional, chrome plated, weight machine workouts that are popular in today's modern gyms. Machine workouts only work on one specific muscle group at a time as opposed to the kettlebell workout which works many muscles at one time. In real life movements such as in carrying groceries, getting out of bed, slamming on the breaks when a car cuts in front of you, and in the martial arts, muscle groups are not isolated. In life's everyday movements, you utilize numerous muscles at the same time and you need balance, flexibility, explosiveness and ballistic power and speed.

Kettlebells are great for the Ageless Warrior, and even better for the athletic Ageless Warrior that still trains in sports and in the martial arts. Kettlebell moves such as swings, snatches, power clean, and presses, are explosive and ballistic just like when you play sports or like in martial arts where you kick, punch, block, throw your opponent, or take him down. These movements work the body in a wide range of angles. It involves the entire body through core stabilization, flexion, extension and rotation in numerous planes. Kettlebells strengthen and condition the martial artist's grip and core. Strength, flexibility, and athletic ability originate in the core of the human body. Great athletes possess great strength, power, and flexibility in the core. Kettlebell training will keep you young, can take you to the next level, and help you achieve your full potential as you age. Kettlebell training will also enhance shoulder rotation, stability, strength, and flexibility to keep you from injuries.

Kettlebells are the perfect training tool for everyone regardless of age. Being compact, kettlebells occupy very little space. With approximately 8x8 feet of space and two kettlebells, you can get a full workout in a short amount of time. You can do a full beginner kettlebell workout in 20 or 30 minutes. Workouts are shorter than weight training, yet they give you an aerobic and anaerobic workout. Shorter workout times give you more free time to enjoy life. You can train with kettlebells as your sole workout since it works strength, muscle tone, cardio and flexibility at the same time. You can also add kettlebells to your existing workout. Before my last back injury, I was training with both kettle bells and weights.

Kettlebells have a rich international history. Kettlebell training, as we know it today, can be traced back to its beginnings in Russia over 300 years ago. Kettlebells have been utilized for athletic and warrior training throughout the world. There is speculation that kettlebells were used by Greek athletes and gladiators thousands of years ago.

Kettlebells were the training tools of choice for the strong men of the early 1900's. The early bodybuilding and muscle building manuals and weight sets all included kettlebells. In the mid-1900's, handles to transform dumbbells to kettlebells came with all weight lifting sets. That is how Bruce Lee began using them. He was ahead of his time in training with kettlebells over 30 years ago. Handles came with the barbell set that he ordered. As per the book, "Bruce Lee, The Art of Expressing the Human Body," Lee trained his back muscles with those kettlebell attachments. John Saxon, co-star of "Enter the Dragon," and martial artist, Dan Inosantos, were introduced to kettlebells by Bruce Lee. Today they continue their kettlebell training.

In the early 1900's, musclemen, bodybuilders and strong men of Europe, Canada and America like Arthur Saxon, Sig Klein, Louis Cyr and Eugen Sandow, to name a few, all trained with kettlebells just like the Russian strongmen and athletes. When kettlebells disappeared in the West, they began to re-flourish in the former Soviet Union. Everyone from common people, those in the military and even Olympic athletes trained with kettlebells. Kettlebells were known to be the USSR secret weapon in their athletic dominance. In 1948, the first kettlebell competition took place in Russia. Later it became Russia's National sport. Thanks to Pavel Tsatsouline, a Russian Kettlebell trainer, kettlebells were reintroduced to the United States.

A military study was done in Russia which compared Kettlebell training against specific forms of physical training. The study divided the participants into two groups. One group only practiced the testing protocol of push-ups, pull ups, a run, a sprint, etc. The other group only lifted kettlebells. In spite of no rehearsal of the testing protocol, the Kettlebell group actually posted better scores in all of these events! That goes to prove that kettlebells truly enhance athletic performance. It's a whole new level of training.

A kettlebell set should consist of 5 to 20 repetitions. When learning and perfecting a move, stay at 5 reps, since with higher reps, fatigue hits and you'll sacrifice form. A kettlebell workout can be classified by 3 types of drills: Ballistic, Grinds, and Hand-to-Hand. Ballistic moves are what make kettlebells unique. They are dynamic and explosive. They help build strength, cardio and endurance. Grinds are the slower pressing moves similar to barbell and dumbbell training even though they are more explosive. Hand-to-Hand moves are similar to juggling. You pass the kettlebell from one hand to the other. This is great for eye-hand coordination, grip training and weapons training.

Kettlebells have grown in popularity in the US. Some are calling it the latest fitness fad. Yet, kettlebell training is not the latest fitness or infomercial fad. They have been around for over 300 years and will surely be around for the next few hundred years.

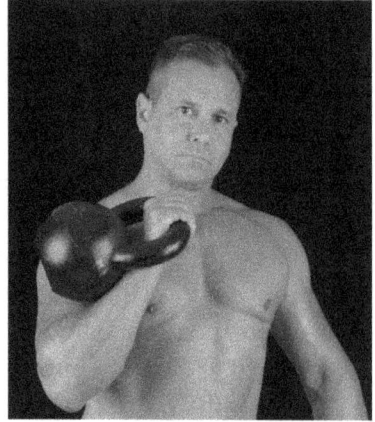

Let me forewarn you. With the growth of kettlebell training and other functional type training, there are many uncertified trainers and personal trainers teaching kettlebell moves incorrectly in gyms, boxes, boot camps, and martial arts studios. Improper kettlebell techniques can cause injuries. Some of the certifications are merely one- or two-day programs. Those trained in such a minimalistic program are unqualified to teach.

When training in different gyms, I have been horrified to see a personal trainer taking their clients through incorrect kettlebell moves. I've even seen videos in top gyms advertising their kettlebell training with terrible form. Do your research and be very careful when looking for a kettlebell trainer.

I'm certified in Hardstyle Kettlebell, Elite Combat Fitness Kettlebell, and Kettlebell Concepts. I have taken Mike Mahler's Kettlebell training, Ageless Body Kettlebell by Andrea Du Cane, and I have also trained in kettlebells in the Action Strength Certification.

Calisthenics

Calisthenics is free weight exercise using your body weight. We all did calisthenics in physical education class in school. I also trained in calisthenics in Marine Corps boot camp and in the Department of Corrections academy. While working as a corrections officer at South Florida Reception Center I noticed that some of the inmates had some of the most muscular and cut up bodies I had ever seen. Most of all they had the best chest development. These inmates had very little weight equipment,

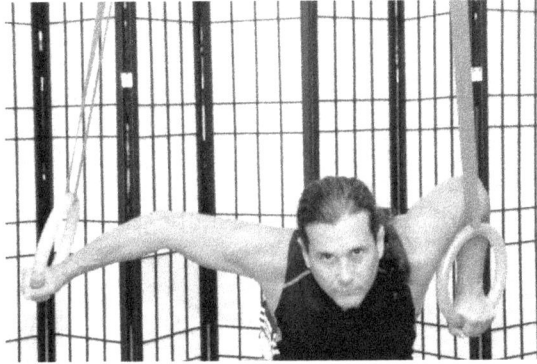

Push-ups on rings 2006

yet they were constantly doing pushups and dips on the hand rails of the stairway.

With your body alone you can build an impressive body. The Russians call it, "The Naked Workout" because you are not using any equipment. With your bodyweight and a pull-up bar you can get a great workout.

Here is a full body beginner's workout using bodyweight exercise and a pull-up bar. You can do this workout three times a week, every other day. You can also do a split routine by splitting it in half and doing each body part two to three times a week. make sure you give each body part at least 48 hours rest. Do thighs, calves, back and biceps on one day and Chest, shoulders, triceps and abdominals on the next day. Your sets and repetitions depend on your fitness level. As you feel better and get in shape you can do abdomens every day.

Thighs: Bodyweight squats or Hindu squats

Calves: Calf Raises

Chest: Pushup

 Regular or different varieties of pushups: Hindu, clapping, traveling, staggered, one arm

Shoulders: Handstand press

Back: Pull-ups (palms of hands away from you)

Biceps: Chin-ups (palms of hands towards you)

Triceps: Diamond pushups (hands under your chest making a diamond shape with your hands)

Abdominals: Leg raises, sit-ups, crunches, dragonfly

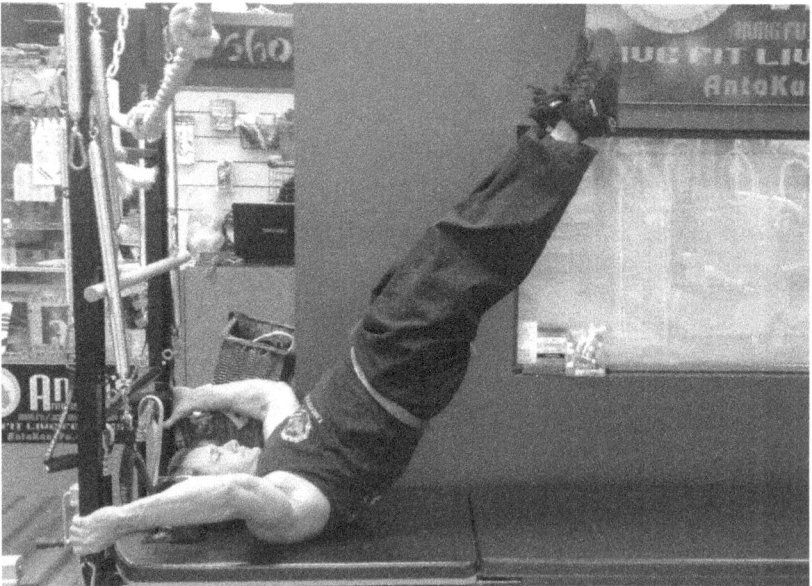

Doing Bruce Lee's Dragonfly for abdominal training at 56 in 2013

Cardiovascular Endurance

Cardiovascular endurance is a super important aspect of fitness, especially as we mature in age. Cardiovascular endurance keeps your heart strong. Keeping your heart strong will keep you healthy and can add years to your life. By keeping the heart strong, you will avoid numerous health problems.

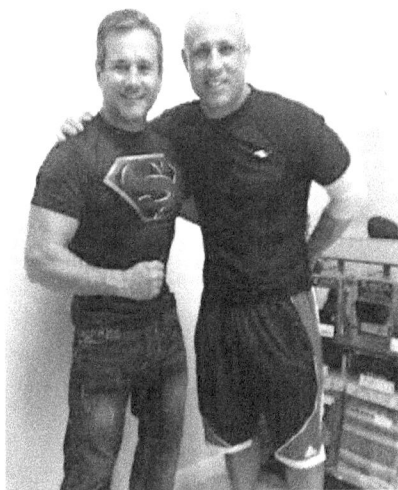

Training Manny Reyes Jr. 40 year old World Karate and Kickboxing Champion and King of the Cage MMA Champion

Your cardio can improve as you age because your heart is a muscle. In the same way that you can build stronger and bigger arms, legs and shoulders, you can also strengthen your heart through cardiovascular training.

You might be surprised at how easy it is to improve your cardiovascular endurance. You can strengthen your heart and get in great shape in only 15 to 20 minutes of interval training, 3 times a week. You can also do one-minute intervals with the battling ropes. You can do Tabatas. A Tabata is doing exercise for 20 seconds and resting 10 seconds for eight sets. After that you can take a short rest period and do another eight sets, exercising for 20 seconds and resting for 10 seconds. You can do Tabatas with bodyweight exercises, martial arts kicks and punches, kettlebells, weights, battling ropes or with any equipment you like.

Beware of Daily High Intensity Workouts

High intensity, heavy weight training with low repetitions is great to build strength and increase testosterone and HGH. Beware of boot camps, CrossFit, and cross training programs that are high repetition, high intensity, and that workout the entire body on a daily bases. This type of training does not let your body recuperate. Remember your muscles need at least 48 hours to rebuild themselves.

As we get older we must train for longevity, build muscle, stay away from injuries, and strengthen our bones. You must be very careful to stay away from these popular cross training types of workouts with high repetition. Stay away from high intensity, high repetition movements especially when those movements involve Olympic lifts and kettlebells. Olympic lifts are hard to learn and were not meant to be done in high repetitions. One of the first rules of kettlebell training is when you are tired or your form gets bad you should put the kettlebell down. This prevents you and others around you from getting hurt.

Stay away from cardio and intense sprints prior to lifting heavy weights. Your technique will suffer and you can get injured. You should not work your entire body without giving it a chance to rest and recuperate.

Those who advocate this high-intensity type of workout have a WOD (workout of the day) which is very challenging, but it doesn't allow your body to recuperate from the previous WOD. Workouts like this overwork your body, which in turn, doesn't allow your muscles to grow to their fullest potential. In such high-intensity workouts, there are usually a lot of injuries that occur, not only with older adults, but even those who are regular athletes can end up with injuries by over-use. They also do a combination of gymnastics, calisthenics, running, sprinting, Olympic lifting, medicine ball training and kettlebells.

The other problem with this type of workout is that you are timed. You write your time on a board and there is constant peer pressure to push yourself harder. You are trying to beat your old score and that of the other members on a daily basis. This competitive spirit is often accompanied with sloppy technique because you are tired and exhausted from pushing yourself to surpass your previous limits and times. Sloppy technique can also lead to further injuries. I've spoken to numerous doctors, physical therapists, and chiropractors, and they all say that over 25% of their clients have been injured doing this type of high-intensity training.

Most of these instructors have only obtained a weekend certification so they do not have the experience or understanding of proper training in all of these exercise modalities.

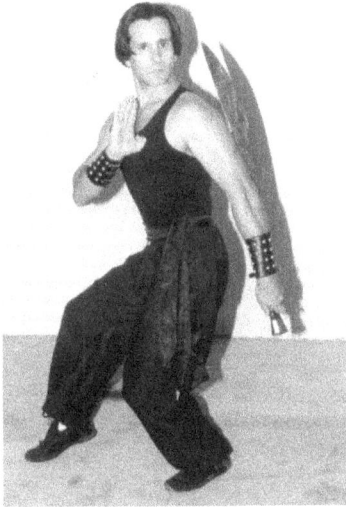

In 1999, 42 years old

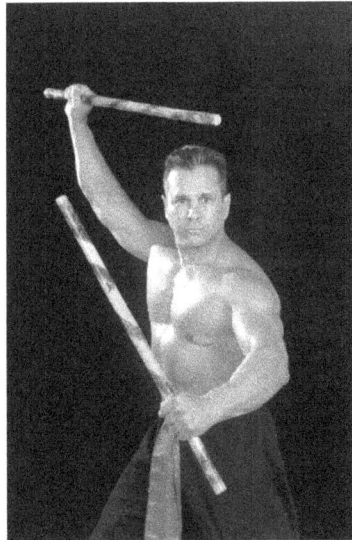

In 2011, 54 years old

Sprints vs Long Distance Training

For years we have heard that you had to do aerobics to lose weight, strengthen your heart and for overall fitness. Today, most fitness experts agree that long periods of cardio or jogging is counterproductive. I remember taking my children to school in the morning and I seeing the dedicated joggers and the members of the local jogging club doing their daily running throughout the neighborhood. One day I had a fitness student ask me if I had noticed how out of shape they looked and the lack of muscle tone that these joggers had. I surely had noticed. If you want to go deeper into this subject just watch an Olympic marathon on TV. Everyone looks frail and sick. Looking at them from the back you cannot tell the difference between the men and the women. The men have lost their wide shoulders and muscles and the women have lost their hips, breasts and shape. Now, let's look at Olympic sprinters both male and female they all have beautiful strong and muscular looking bodies. Running long distance is not a natural act. Our bodies were not made for long distance running or an hour of aerobics.

As we age it is a fact that we tend to lose muscle mass. If we workout smartly we can build muscle as we age. Just like a sprinter, Short Burst Intense Interval Training is the best way to strengthen your heart and not lose muscle.

Have you noticed that the people that spend the most time on treadmills, in aerobic classes, and in any form of endurance training and especially running, do not look good? Endurance training does very little to help the age reversal process. Long duration exercise routines accelerate the aging process by increasing free radicals. Free radicals destroy muscularity. As we age, we start losing muscle and consequently, this is very counterproductive.

The risk for sudden cardiac death is much higher for long-distance runners than it is for any other type of athlete. The best way to strengthen your heart is with intensity rather than long distance running or long duration exercise. As natural hunters, our bodies were made for short intervals such as chasing down the prey. Short burst of intense exercise followed by a short rest such as high intensity sprinting will get you in great shape.

Today we know that doing nonstop aerobics for an hour or more will not help you increase your long capacity or strengthen your heart. In studies at Laval University in Quebec, Canada, they compared short burst intense exercise to traditional cardio. In the study they had the cyclist do 45 minutes without stopping. They had another group do brief 90 second intense bursts. The people doing the cardio burned more calories yet, the group that trained for 90 second lost more body fat.

High intensity interval training such as sprinting will help boost your testosterone and HGH levels. Slow one-hour jogging or an hour of aerobic exercise will not have an effect in raising testosterone or HGH. That's one of the reasons that sprinters have muscular bodies.

Long duration aerobics and jogging can cause knee and joint problems. By no means am I condoning being a coach potato and not exercising. There are better ways to train then by jogging or aerobics. Yet, if you enjoy running it is better to run than to be an overweight coach potato.

To start your sprinting program, you can sprint for a block and then walk back at a slow pace to bring your heart rate back to normal. The amount of times you do this will depend on your fitness level. If you have not exercised for a while, start with 3 laps and build up to 5. Each lap you should go faster and with more intensity.

I rarely do traditional cardio training. My cardio comes from boxing or kickboxing training. Usually 3-minute rounds with a 1-minute rest. At times, due to my back injuries, I do 20 minutes on the treadmill. I walk fast for 2 minutes and sprint for 1 minute. I finish the routine with a 45-second sprint and a 30-second sprint. To get in great shape, lose fat, build muscle, and stay healthy, you must workout with intensity.

I believe that there is an exception to every rule and I will breakthe rules. As much as I dislike long distance running, I

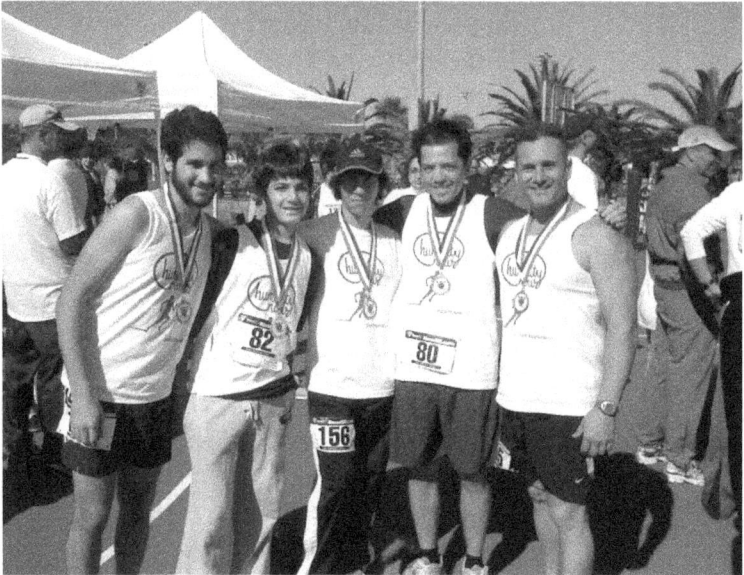

Humility Now/Anta's Fitness and Self Defense 5K Team 2010

have to budge for my family. In 2010, my son, Julio David, asked me to train with him to do a 5 K run. So, we put a team together from our martial arts fitness center and his non-profit organization "Humility Now." Our small team did great. Five out of seven of our team members placed in their divisions. Julio and Jon-Paul (my two sons) and I took third place. We had one student place second and another other student placed third.

86

Battling Ropes

Battling Ropes is taking the fitness industry by storm. It is a low impact workout. It's great for mature adults since it doesn't bother your knees or joints. This type of training is getting so popular that you can see it in sports drink commercials. It is being used by numerous football teams, United States Olympic Wrestling Team, UFC fighters, Special Forces, Federal Agents, Olympians, College and Pro-Athletes. You might have seen Battling Ropes on TV in previews of UFC champions and fighters in training preparing for their fights. You can also see Battling Ropes on TUF (The Ultimate Fighter) TV show. Even celebrities and the Hollywood elite are now incorporating rope training into their training routines. Kim Kardashian is a believer of hardcore rope training and her trainer, trainer of the stars, Gunner Petterson, is training the Hollywood elite with ropes. No, we are not talking about jumping rope. This new type of rope workout is redefining interval and cardio training.

Rope training is a unique, functional aerobic and anaerobic, no-impact training system done with 1 1/2 to 2 inch ropes that measure 50 to 100 feet in length with unique names such as Tsunami and the Wave. To get started you need to wrap a

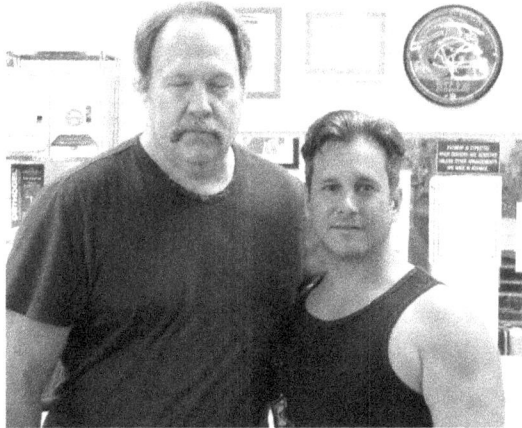

Getting certified in Battling Ropes with John Brooksfield 2009

rope around a pole or tie it to a heavy object like a kettlebell. You then grasp the ends of the rope and begin to move the ropes to make waves, circles, and other specific moves. When doing waves, the objective is to use velocity to sustain the waves all the way to the end of the pole. With shorter ropes such as 30- or 40-foot ropes, you can grab the ends and use them without having to wrap them around anything. You can also use a partner on the other end of the rope instead of a pole or heavy object.

If you do not have a rope you can do some of the moves with a beach towel. You can grab the towel by one end and make waves. If you prefer to do it with a partner it will make it even harder. You can grab one end of a towel and your partner grabs the other end. Simultaneously you both make waves. Just 20 to 30 seconds of this will raise your heart rate. So now you have no excuse for not training while on vacation. When I was a recruit in the United States Marine Corps in Parris Island, South Carolina we used to dust our blankets using this method. What we did was to have a recruit on each side of the large blanket, shaking and making waves. This was an incredible cardio and upper body workout which pumped and burned your triceps.

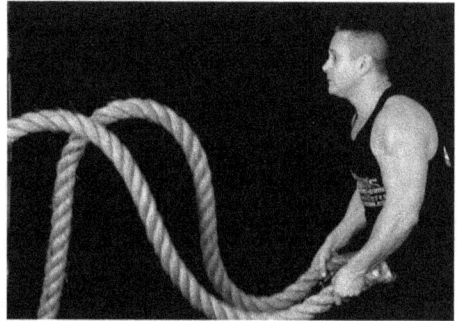

What makes Battling Ropes training fun and unique is that there are so many ways in which you can train with them. For strength, endurance, and grip strength training you can use the pole system with the ropes. In the pole system you wrap a 100 feet of rope once or twice around a pole and then pull the rope to the end of the pole. You can pull the rope while standing, sitting, or on your knees. This system of rope training works your muscles in a different way than when sustaining waves.

Regardless if you're handicapped, a sedentary coach potato, a novice or elite world-class athlete this new and exciting rope workout will tax your entire system in a short time of 60 seconds or less. Your core will be absolutely trashed after 60 seconds of the power surge that these ropes demand. Working out with ropes will enable you to maintain power, strength and explosiveness over a greater period of time to perform at your highest level for a much longer time in the sport of your choice.

 Are you ready to lose weight, get stronger, and get in the best shape of your life? Then get ready for Battling Rope fitness. Your gains of strength, stamina, and power will be mind-blowing. Fitness training with ropes is a no-impact, high-velocity, pure adrenal surge functional training workout! Before training with ropes, I had never experienced a cardio workout at this level. A rope training system is a functional, highly effective form of training and conditioning for athletes or anyone wanting to get in great shape fast. Battling Ropes training drills will help improve your grip strength, improve your ability to increase power and sustain that power output for longer periods of time. It will also improve your aerobic and anaerobic capacity, teach the muscles of the entire body to work together to maximize performance, and add a fun new twist to your workout.

The great thing is that you can do rope training by yourself or with a partner. You can do it at your home, gym, martial arts center or at the park. You can do it as your sole workout or you can combine them with any other training tool you like such as calisthenics, kettlebells, barbells, dumbbells, sand bags, medicine balls, and Indian clubs, or with plyometric exercises. This is such an intense workout that I'm sure that most physically fit people will have a hard time sustaining a wave for 30 or 40 seconds. There are hundreds of moves that you can do, but the staple of this rope routine is making different types of waves or undulations.

I began training with ropes in March, 2009, when I became certified in Battling Ropes by its creator, John Brookfield, which took place at my good friend, Frank Dimeo's, training center. We were the first two trainers certified in "Battling Ropes" in the state of Florida by its originator, John Brookfield. Frank was the first in central Florida and I was the first trainer in South Florida to be certified in Battling Ropes.

Benefits of Battling Ropes Training

No impact cardio workout
Intense core workout
Get in the best shape of your life while rehabbing injuries
Increase maximum heart rates in minutes
Increase power and speed, which equal velocity
Increase aerobic and anaerobic capacity
Increase your motivation and mental endurance
Increase power and strength
Increase athletic ability
Increase your body's ability to burn fat

Today, most gyms have Battling Ropes, yet I rarely see anyone doing them correctly. I've even seen some Olympians and UFC Fighters do it incorrectly. The good thing is that even if you do it wrong, it is still very hard to get injured. One of the best videos of Battling Ropes I've seen was with Brock Lesner, the WWE and UFC Champion. What made it exceptionally remarkable was that Brock was using 2-inch ropes which are incredibly difficult to move. I highly recommend Battling Ropes for the Ageless Warrior.

Flexibility and Mobility

Flexibility and mobility are similar, but they are not the same.
Flexibility is your ability to move statically. Joint mobility is
being able to move a limb through the full range of motion.
I've been stretching all my life due to my martial arts training.
I started doing joint mobility exercises less than a year ago
after hosting a joint mobility workshop at my training center
with my friend, Eric Guttman.

All martial art stylists agree that posture and spinal flexibility is
of the utmost importance. A healthy spine is bendable and
flexible. Chinese martial arts use the analogy of a bamboo
plant to describe Kung Fu and Tai Chi. Bamboo is not as thick
or as wide as an oak tree or most other trees. Yet when
Hurricane Andrew destroyed parts of South Florida, a bamboo
farm was untouched. Bamboo is hard, yet soft (Ying and Yang).
A bamboo tree stems from strong roots. Its characteristics are
tall, straight, and strong sprouts. When the wind blows,
bamboo can flow and bend. Your spine should be flexible
enough to bend like bamboo and still stay firm and strong.
Pilates is your key to spinal flexibility.

Tai Chi master and Chinese medicine doctor Cheng Man-Ching
advised Tai Chi practitioners, "Make your spine upright as a
string of pearls that does not lean". In Pilates they also use an
analogy of a pearl necklace to describe articulating your spine,
one vertebrate at a time. I have also heard traditional
instructors say that if you practice 1000 times, then correct
body posture will eventually become natural.

Stretching

Stretching is an essential part of any fitness program. It is also the most neglected. Most people will do aerobic and anaerobic training, yet very few will implement a stretching routine in their physical fitness program. There is a correct way and an incorrect way to stretch. The proper way to stretch is static stretching. Static stretching is holding the stretch for 10 to 30 seconds. Most people including coaches, martial arts instructors, and dance and gymnastics instructors wrongly teach stretching in a ballistic type of bouncing. Bouncing can damage your ligaments and tighten your muscles. Make sure that your body is warmed up before you stretch by jumping rope, running in place or shuffling. It is also good to stretch at the end of a physical workout. It will help reduce lactic acid build up to alleviate the post workout pain.

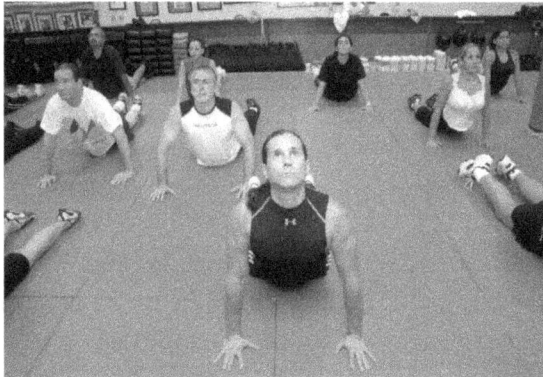

Cooling down in the XFT (Xtreme Functional Training) class at the end of the workout 2006

Stretching will make your muscles longer and, bigger. A flexible muscle will help you avoid injuries. Regularly implementing stretching into your workout routine will not only make your muscles bigger, but stronger and more flexible.

Indian Clubs for Circular Strength

No other exercise modalities can give you the shoulder joint mobility and circular strength of Indian Clubs. If I would have known and trained with Indian Clubs in my younger days, I would have never have had shoulder injuries or dislocations.

Indian Clubs or Swing Bells, as they are also called, were introduced to America in the 1800's. They are made out of wood and resemble bowling pins or juggling clubs. They come in different sizes and weights depending on your experience, strength and your objective. You can use them for rehab or for strength gains and raw power. Working out with Indian Clubs might be described as Circular Weight Training. It develops rotary and angular or diagonal strength. Indian Club Training will increase stability and prevent injury in the shoulder region. You'll feel your shoulder muscles getting stronger and more flexible. This is an excellent exercise for Ageless Warriors.

The club is the oldest and most ancient of all weapons. When we think of pre-historic man we immediately think of the brawny caveman dragging his weapon of choice the club. The club evolved into a highly sophisticated martial arts weapon used worldwide by most ancient cultures at one time or another. Many cultures used the club, not only for fighting, but also to strengthen the warrior's body. Modern Club Swinging has its roots in India and Persia (modern day Iran and Iraq). In India they referred to their clubs as Gadas and Karelas. In Persia they were known as Meels. In the late 18th century, the British that occupied India were amazed by the strength and power of Indian slaves and police officers. Thereafter, they took the ancient tool/weapon to Britain and named them Indian Clubs.

You will find the idea of clubs mentioned in numerous religions. In the Old Testament, Cain murdered his brother, Abel, with a club. The Greek/Roman mythological demi-god, Hercules, was worshiped for his power and strength. He was known for his skills with the bow and arrow and the club. In

India, the club, or Gada as they call it, is a symbol of invincibility and physical power. Almost every God or Goddess in the Hindu religion is pictured holding a Gada. From ancient Persian strongmen to the famous Indian wrestler, The Great Gama, to turn of the last century strongman to British and American physical culture in the 1800's and early 1900's, Indian Club have been used to create a definitive edge in health, strength, and fitness. Today even five-time Ultimate Fighting World Champion, Pat Miletich, trains with Indian Clubs. Pat has trained more world champions than any other trainer in the world and has been voted the number one trainer in the world for two years in a row.

Sim D. Kehoe produced the first clubs in the USA and was also the person most responsible for the growth of Club Swinging in America at the end of the 19th century. In the late 19th century a movement called "Muscular Christianity" popularized Club Swinging. This movement linked physical training to moral and spiritual development. Club Swinging was also popularized by strong man acts, professional wrestlers, and athletes from around the world. Indian Clubs were endorsed by American Presidents, Ulysses S. Grant and Teddy Roosevelt, and also by Queen Victoria of England. Club Swinging was popular as a means of fitness and sport that a series of Club Swinging tobacco cards (similar to baseball cards) were printed.

Club Swinging became an Olympic sport. It was called "Rhythmic Gymnastics" in the St. Louis Olympics of 1904 in which the Americans won all of the divisions. It continued in the Olympics until the 1932 Los Angeles Olympics in which the Americans won all of the divisions again. Club Swinging was once practiced in many colleges, gymnasiums, the military, and in social clubs throughout America. It was a very popular women's activity in primary through secondary schools. Many colleges and girls' clubs had competition and demonstration teams. Many gyms and PE programs had Indian

Clubs for boys so that they could develop into masculine strong young men.

Through the efforts of Dr. Ed Thomas and his brother Dick, Club Swinging is resurfacing today. I've had the privilege to train and get certified by Dr. Ed Thomas as an Indian Club

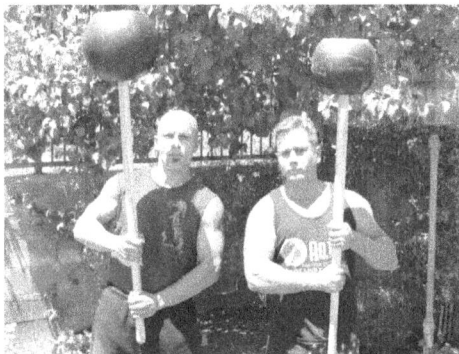

Gada Training with Harinder Singh

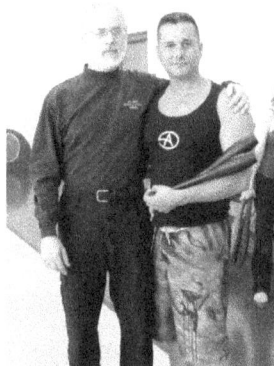

Getting certified by Dr Ed Thomas 2010

Specialist at the first Indian club certification by Dragon Door. My studio, Anta's Fitness and Self Defense in Miami (Doral), Florida, is proud to be a pioneer in modern Indian Club swinging. We began one of the first group and children Indian Club classes in the nation. Our studio is fully equipped with Indian Clubs for children and adult

Tai Chi/Qi Gong

Tai Chi or taiji is short for t'ai chi ch'uan or tàijíquán in America. Tai chi ch'uan translates to "supreme ultimate fist, boundless fist, supreme ultimate boxing or great extremes boxing." Tai Chi is an internal Chinese martial art practiced for its health benefits, yet it is also a combative art. There are five traditional schools of Tai Chi: Chen, Yang, Wu (Hao), Wu, and Sun.

It is very common to see hundreds of people practicing Tai Chi and Qi Gong in parks in China. There is evidence through medical research that Tai Chi is helpful in improving general health for older people. The slow martial arts moves will help you relax, relieve stress, and help attain balance which is extremely important as we age.

Tai Chi is practiced as a graceful form of exercise. It involves a series of movements performed in a slow, focused manner and accompanied by deep breathing. Tai Chi is low- impact exercise. It puts minimal stress on muscles and joints, making it safe for anyone regardless of fitness level or age. It is suitable for older adult who otherwise may not exercise.

I am not a Tai Chi or Qi Gong instructor. I have been doing some simple Qi Gong moves that I learned from my Jeet Kune Do instructor. Yes, Jeet Kune Do, Bruce Lee's art. Bruce Lee's first martial art was Tai Chi which his father taught him.

Many years ago I learned the Yang Short form and after that I learned a short version of a Cheng Tai Chi form. After I stopped practicing due to the other martial arts I have studied, I forgot those forms. I have been planning to add more Qi Gong and Tai Chi to my training program for years. My wife has been pushing me to start Tai Chi training again. Since I have a hyper, type-A personality, Tai Chi helps me relax. So, I recently started studying Tai Chi at the park.

Pilates

Pilates is great for flexibility, joint mobility and strengthening of the core. In 1999, I was certified in Pilates. I stopped teaching and training in Pilates many years ago, but at times, I'll add some Pilate's moves to my stretching routine. My wife is a fully certified Pilate's mat and equipment instructor and teaches it at our center, Anta's Fitness and Self Defense. My daughter-in-law, Kathryn Anta, is also a fully certified Pilate's instructor in New York City. I know that eventually I'll get back to doing more Pilates.

Pilates was developed around 100 years ago by a great innovator, Joseph H. Pilates (1880-1967). He was a German immigrant of Greek decent. At 87, the age he died, he was in robust health, and exercised daily. Who knows how much longer he would have lived if he would not have succumbed to the effects of smoke inhalation, due to the fire that destroyed his studio.

My fascination with Pilates began in 1999, shortly after I was certified in Pilates mat work, when I noticed the similarities of Joseph Pilates' childhood and my own.. Joseph was a small and sickly child who suffered from asthma, rickets and rheumatic

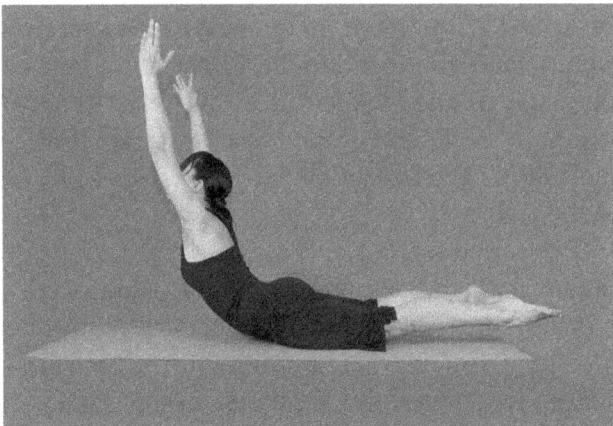

Elena Anta Pilates

97

fever. As an adult, he later became a boxer and taught self-defense. He studied both Eastern and Western forms or exercise including Yoga, Zen and ancient Greek and Roman regiments. He put it all together to help WWII soldiers recuperating from wounds and injuries. His greatest accomplishment was in developing numerous and unusual kinds of exercise equipment. The Pilates equipment being used today is identical to what Pilates originated. He developed his first apparatus from a hospital bed; later in NY, he began physical therapy for injured ballet dancers. Today, Pilates is practiced by many celebrities including Cameron Diaz, Sandra Bullock, Madonna, Kate Hudson, Hilary Duff, Reese Witherspoon, Daisy Fuentes, Vanessa Williams, Patrick Swayze, Bill Murray, Danny Glover, Glen Close, Melanie Griffin, Minnie Driver, Jennifer Aston, Jennifer Beals, Joan Collins, Sigoney Weaver and Gregory Peck, to name a few.

Pilates is much more than an exercise method. Joseph Pilates developed his program to create a healthy body, a healthy mind, and a healthy life with balance. He blended many disciplines together to restore harmony and balance on three levels; physical, mental, and spiritual. Originally, he referred to his work as "Contrology" because he believed that the mind controls the body, and the spirit builds the body. He dedicated his life's work to helping others achieve their full potential in life. He passed his methods on to his students and disciples who, in turn, carried them into the 21st century, impacting the lives of people all over the world. Pilates must be rolling in his grave as these weekend-certified instructors are destroying his lifelong study of the human body by incorrectly teaching Pilates.

You cannot learn Pilates properly by a video or an untrained fitness instructor. I've seen some good videos on Pilates; but I have also seen videos where a fitness instructor with very little knowledge in Pilates is breaking every Pilates rule and principle. Even a good video cannot correct your alignment, technique or breathing. A well-rounded Pilate's program will take the spine through its full range of motion. These movements will keep the discs nourished and healthy. Pilates strengthens the muscles that

support the spine and increases its flexibility therefore reducing compression and pain. Pilates will help you reeducate the body and develop healthier postural habits. It will strengthen the muscles that support

the spine. A balanced muscle is both flexible and strong. Your muscle groups also need to have a balance in their relationship with one another for optimum health and fitness. Pilates will do all this and more. Before starting Pilates classes check the instructor's certification and hours of study. My wife and I have both seen people teaching

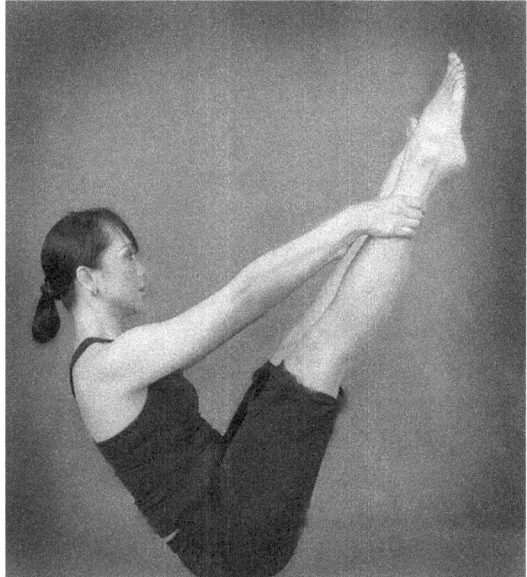

Pilates in chain health spas with a weekend certification or with no certification at all. I remember when my wife, Elena, went to an LA Fitness to tryout a Pilate's class. The class looked more like a stretching abdominal class with just a few Pilates moves done incorrectly. At the end of the class the instructor came up to her and asked her how long she had been doing Pilates. When she told her she was an instructor the lady asked her for advice and confessed that she was not certified.

Yoga

My wife also cross trains in Yoga. I have gone a few times with her to do a Yoga class and it has truly alleviated my chronic back pain. Restorative Yoga is my favorite. You hold the Yoga positions for a longer time in a relaxing technique.

Yoga is an ancient, mind, body, and spirt workout which originated in India around 300 BC. You learn to utilize your diaphragm when breathing. When doing Yoga you will learn to relax and treat your body with care and respect. By doing Yoga you will be improving your circulation, becoming more flexible, and strengthening your core.

Yoga is not just about stretching. Stretching and joint mobility is certainly involved, but Yoga is about creating balance in the body by developing greater strength and flexibility. You'll develop strength and flexibility by holding certain poses and postures.

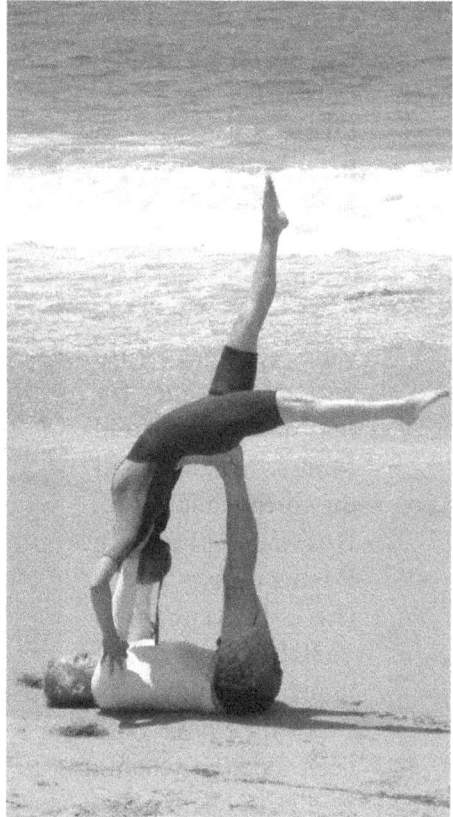

Jen and Kerry Yoga at the Beach

As this book was being edited, I made a decision to stop my boxing and Tai Chi training to add Yoga to relieve back pain and to also strengthen my back.

Balance

Having good balance is of upmost important to the Ageless Warrior. As we age, numerous physiological changes take place. Loss of balance and falls increases. Balance exercise help reduce the risk of falls and fractures. Health care cost associated with falls is astonishing for the older adult.

Performing balance exercises on an unstable surface is the key to balance. There are many ways to attain balance and keep our balance as we age. Martial arts, BOSU and physio ball moves are my exercise of choice for balance.

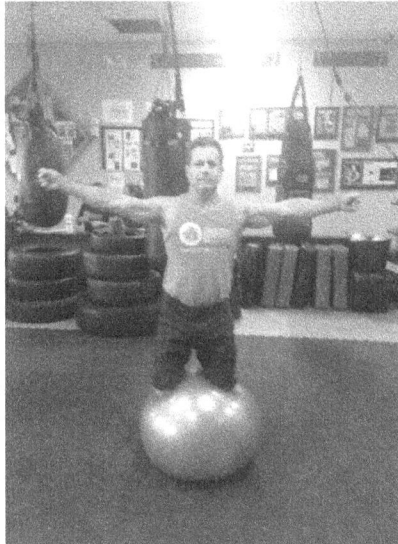

The younger you start working on balance exercise the better. I was blessed to have trained steadily and seriously in balance in my thirties when studying kung fu. If you don't have good balance, don't despair. You can still enhance your balance at any age. You need to take time to check your balance. If you find yourself using handrails when taking stairs, then that is one sign that you need to start balance training. If you have to sit down to tie your shoes that is also a sign of poor balance.

There are many things that you can do to improve your balance. Walk on different surfaces when you can. When at a park alternate walking on the pavement and on grass. At the beach take a stroll walking on the sand, better yet run on the sand. Running on the sand strengthens your calves, thighs, feet and ankles. Walk up and down stairs without holding on to the rails. When you feel comfortable and have the balance and endurance, start running up and down the stairs. Do calf raises with your body weight and or with weights or calf machines.

You can stand on a BOSU ball alternating legs. A BOSU ball looks like half ball on a platform. This dome-like exercise tool allows you to use the half ball on a flat surface while giving you a rounded surface to improve your balance.

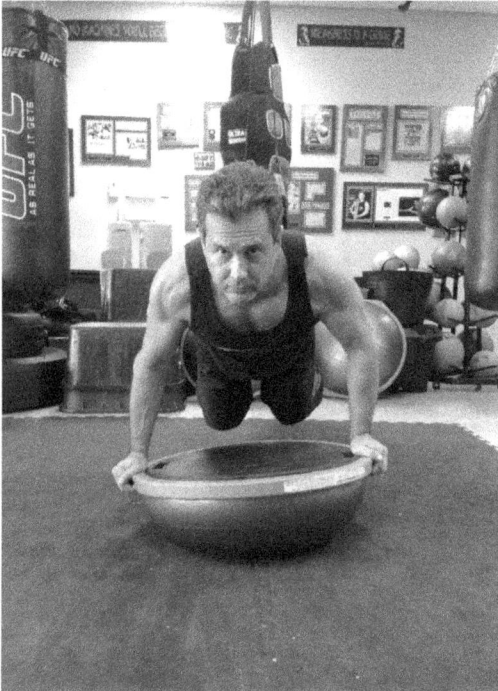

BOSU Ball pushups with feet hanging on Airfit in 2013

There are also numerous balancing exercises you can do on a physic ball. These are harder to do than on a BOSU ball. Make sure you do any balance exercise on a physic ball over a mat or on grass, for your safety.

Another exercise that I think has helped me with my balance is grabbing things with my toes. When I was a kid in elementary school I had a teacher tell us that with time humans would evolve and start losing their toes since we did not use them. I think that I was traumatized and started picking up things with my toes. Even though I do not believe in evolution, I still try to pick up things with my toes. When you do this while standing up, you will be balancing on one leg.

Martial Arts Great for Balance

I believe that I have good balance at 57 years old. They say that at around 50 you start do lose your balance. I feel that due to my martial arts training I have retained my balance. In kung fu, we work numerous stances and many moves up on one leg. This gives you great balance and strengthens your ankles. All martial arts kick and have kicking drills. When you kick you are also sustaining your body on one leg which is great balance. In Muay Thai kickboxing, when you kick, you lift the heel of the supporting leg off the ground. This type of kicking and training will give you even better balance and it also strengthens your ankles. Another way to enhance your balance is through boxing, kickboxing or Jeet Kune Do footwork.

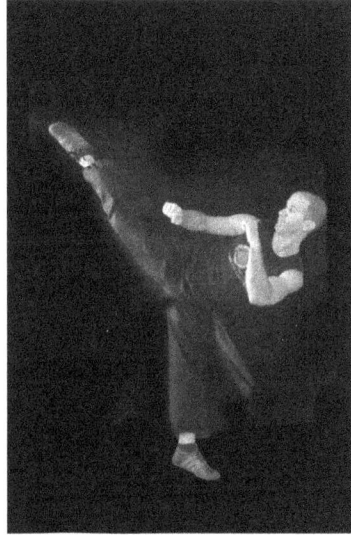

Hector Arcia kicking

Here are some drills to enhance your balance and strengthen your ankles.

Kung Fu Drills: Lifting one leg for balance and kicking will help your balance since you are on one leg.

Crane Stance: Stand on your right leg, lift the left leg, bending at the knee, and hold it horizontal. Bring your right arm up high with the palm of your hand facing the roof or what the Chinese call holding the heavens. Your left arm is down with your palm facing down or what the Chinese call pushing the earth. Hold it for as long as you can and then switch and do the other side.

T-Kick: Stand on one leg. Without bringing your leg down, do a front kick, back kick and side kick. Then switch legs and repeat.

Side Step Jump Shifting from Cat Stance: Get into a cat stance. In a cat stance, you should have 3/4 of your weight on the back leg. On the front leg, lift your heel off the ground and keep only a quarter of your weight on the toes of your front leg. Imagine that you are on a train track and you have to jump to the other side of the track. When you jump, end up on the opposite side with the other leg in front.

Muay Thai Kickboxing Drills
In Muay Thai, all your kicks and knees are done on your toes with heels off the ground. Lifting your heels off the ground will work your balance even more than regular kicking. Not only are you balancing on one leg, but your toes are holding your weight.

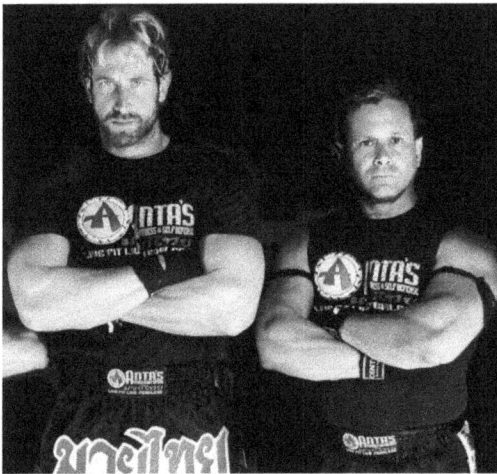
With Muay Thai student Spanish Actor Gabriel Soto 39 years old

Shadow Boxing on Tires: Stand on a tire move around the tire as you shadow Muay Thai box. It is very hard to keep your balance, especially when you kick.

Pad Work on Tires: Stand on a tire move around the tire while your trainer or partner feeds you Muay Thai pad combinations.

My injuries

I started martial arts at the age of 13, and began serious bodybuilding at 18 years old. Since I was 18, I've worked out with weights, martial arts or other fitness modalities. From the beginning, the road was not easy. I had to train around numerous injuries and maladies.

While in high school, one kid that wrestled found out I had trained in Judo while in Jr. High. We started grappling and I felt that he had injured my shoulder. After that, I always felt tightness in that shoulder. You might ask, "Which shoulder was it?" I can't remember since after that both shoulders were injured.

When I first started working out at the age of 18, I was battling sciatica. I spent years working out my upper body, but not my legs. Yeah, I looked pretty funny, having built a muscular upper body with bird legs. I was so self-conscious that I would even go to the beach wearing long pants.

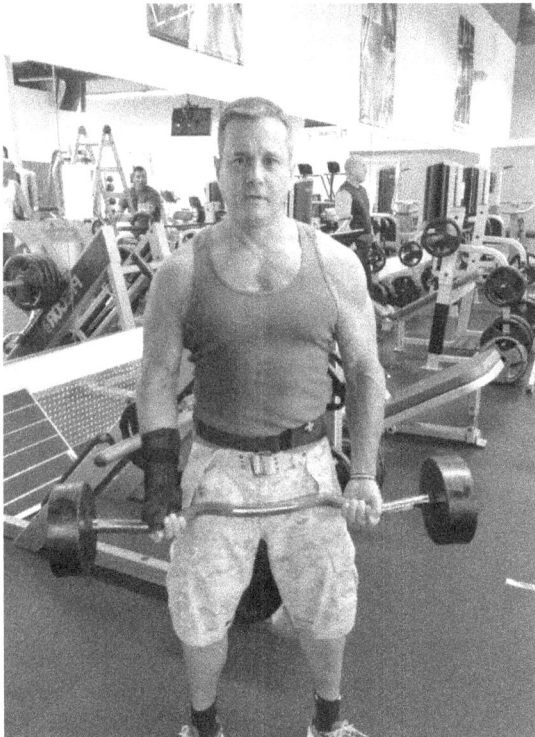

I trained with injured hand until the day of the operation 2013

When I went to Marine Corps boot camp in December of 1980,

my sciatic pain went away. I just might have been too stressed out to think about it.

After boot camp, I began bodybuilding again, but this time I started doing legs also. One day when I was talking about competing, a friend told me that I could never win due to my bird legs. This is what finally motivated me to begin training my legs seriously. At that time, I was not able to do barbell squats due to my back problem. I build my legs by doing heavy hack squats and leg presses. I also stretched a lot since it relieved my back pain. I used to love breaking the stereotype and myth that bodybuilders were muscle bound. I was able to do a full split. I was also able to bend over with legs straight and touch the ground with the palms of my hands. I was also able to sit with my legs open and touch my chest to the floor. This would freak out all of the skeptics that could not believe that a bodybuilder was flexible.

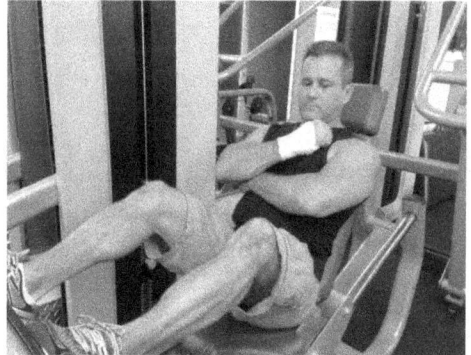

Working out the day after trigger finger surgery on thumb in 2013

My competitive bodybuilding days ended after dislocating both shoulders at a Karate tournament in 1986. I had trained in Judo in Jr high school. In high school I had trained in kung fu, karate, and kenpo. It was in my senior year in high school that I stopped martial arts training to focus on bodybuilding. After years of bodybuilding, I decided to combine my bodybuilding with martial arts training. I went to a tournament and in a sparring match I partially dislocated both shoulders. It was my fault because, with my adrenaline pumping, I started throwing incorrect and wild punches. First, I dislocated one shoulder and then I continued fighting and dislocated the other shoulder. The real pain did not even hit me until after the match was finished. I've always had to train around injuries. I had to train around shoulder injuries, neck and back problems, tendonitis around the elbows, pain under my thumbs, finger injuries. I also made it through hepatitis, vertigo, and gout. Some of these injuries and medical problems stopped me completely from training, but with others, I just continued training around them.

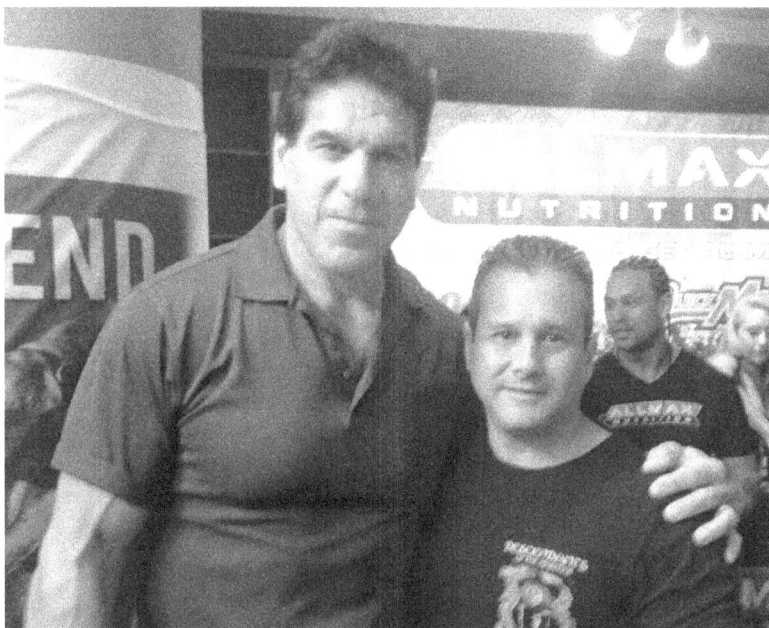

With Lou "The Incredible Hulk" Ferrigno 2012

Everyone has some deficiencies, mental or physical. Lou Ferrigno won the Mr. America and Mr. Universe titles and well known for his role in the original *"Incredible Hulk"* TV series. While he was competing in Donald Trumps, *"The Apprentice,"* some of his teammates said he was the weakest link due to his disability. Lou got very upset and replied "Everyone has a disability." Lou became deaf as a small child and he is right. There is no excuses. You should train around injuries. I remember Billy Blank in the Tae Bo infomercials saying, "Where there's a will there's a way."

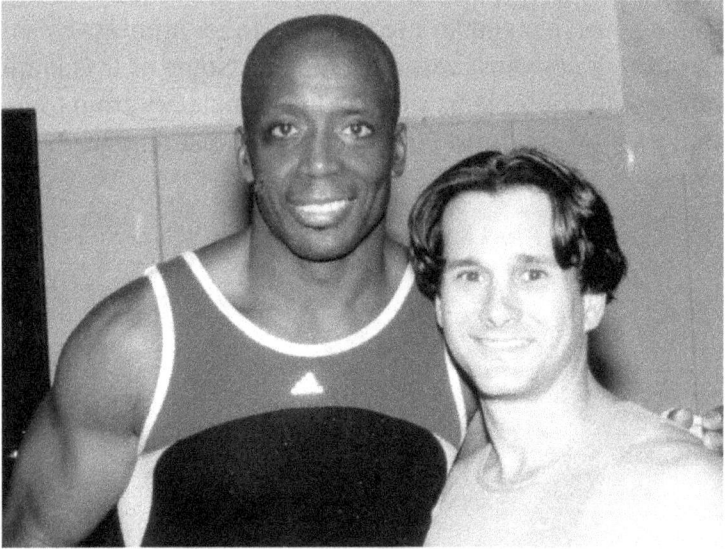

Training with Billy Blanks Tae Bo 1999

One of the great things that I've learned in the Marine Corps is "Adapt, Improvise and Overcome" which is similar to Bruce Lee's concept of "Adapt what is useful, reject what is useless and make it your own." For over 25 years, I could not do barbell bench press due to my shoulder injuries. I adapted by doing machines or dumbbells for chest. For the last four to five months, I've been doing barbell bench press. I bring the bar as far down to the chest as I can without feeling pain and most of the time the bar will not touch my chest.

For my back problems I hang from a pull-up bar. I hang from an inversion table. I use a hard roller similar to a foam roller yet shorter and harder on my back to work trigger points. I also use a lacrosse ball on my back, hips, and shoulders as a trigger point massage. I stretch and do joint mobility exercises.

Staying Fit while on Vacation

You don't have to gain weight and get out of shape while on vacation. One of my favorite things to do is to find a gym while on vacation. I've trained in gyms in hotels, on cruises, and in different cities around the world. I've trained on cruises in the Caribbean and in Mediterranean. In hotels in Rome, Dominican Republic, Columbia, and in numerous states of the U.S., I've trained in terrible hotel gyms and in some great ones also. I've

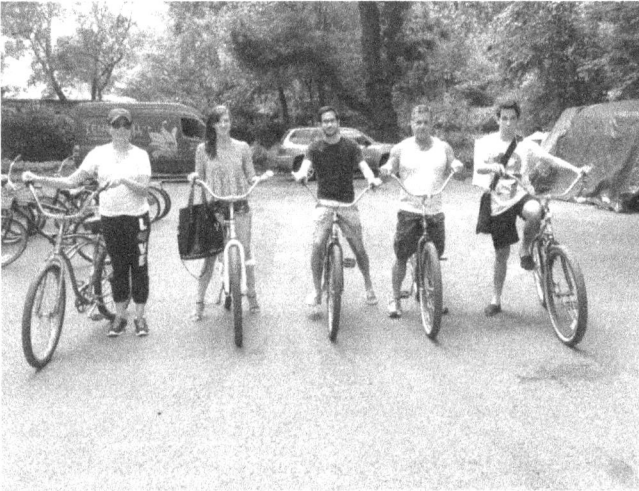

On vacation visiting our son Julio and his wife in NY. Bike riding in Central Park 2013

jogged in the streets of Cartagena, Columbia, and in Manhattan, New York, just to name a few. I've hiked through mountains in Colorado and in North Carolina.

As I write this book my wife and I celebrated our 25th wedding anniversary in Europe and finished the trip by visiting or son in New York. The first thing my wife and I did when we got to Rome was to workout in the hotel's gym. It wasn't one of the best facilities we've worked out in, but we improvised. After spending two and a half days in Rome, we went on a Mediterranean cruise. The cruise ship had a fairly decent gym. I worked out every day in Rome, took one day off in the cruise due to back injury, and then took one day off in New York. I usually train five to six days a week. In the three weeks that we were in Europe and New York, I trained three weeks straight, taking only two days off.

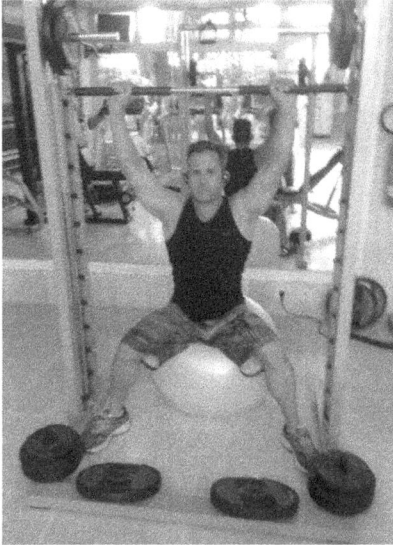

First thing I did when I arrived in Rome after a long plane trip was workout May 2014

Being muscular is a great conversation starter. I once heard a smoker say that smokers are friendlier people. Since they have to smoke outside of buildings with other smokers, they talk and get to know each other. I also once heard someone tell me that his tattoos have helped start conversations because people would ask him about his tattoos. For me there is no better conversation starter than having a muscular body, especially overseas. It is ironic to think that someone is willing to endanger their health and contract cancer by smoking cigarettes for conversation. I don't think that smoking or tattoos would have given me the attention that a muscular body gave me. That's not too bad for someone who is constantly getting mail from AARP, right?.

Let me tell you about my experience in Europe. While training at the gym on the cruise, I re-injured my back while throwing myself back on a bench with heavy dumbbells. That night I had a massage and started taking anti-inflammatory medication. I only had a few pills left, but I was able to purchase more medication at a pharmacy in Turkey. What I paid for them there was actually less than what the normal copayment on my insurance plan! In Turkey and Europe and in most countries around the world, you do not need a prescription for medication like this and it is super inexpensive.

I noticed that in Europe there were not many muscular people. In my stops in Italy, Greece, and in Turkey, I only noticed one person that wasn't a tourist that looked like he worked out with weights. In general, though, they look like they are in better shape than the average American. There were very little overweight people in Italy, Greece and Turkey.

There are no language barriers when you are muscular. I felt like a celebrity when getting off at ports in the Mediterranean. In Italy, I had people flex muscles and call me "fisico culturista" which translates to "bodybuilder" in English. In Greece, I was called "Hercules" and "Leonidas" (the Spartan King). Turkey, I was asked if I was a bodybuilder and was also constantly called "Rambo." It's funny, because I was called Rambo in Jamaica also. I guess that people associate muscular Americans with Rambo in some countries. In the same trip to Europe, we also stopped to see our eldest son and his wife who

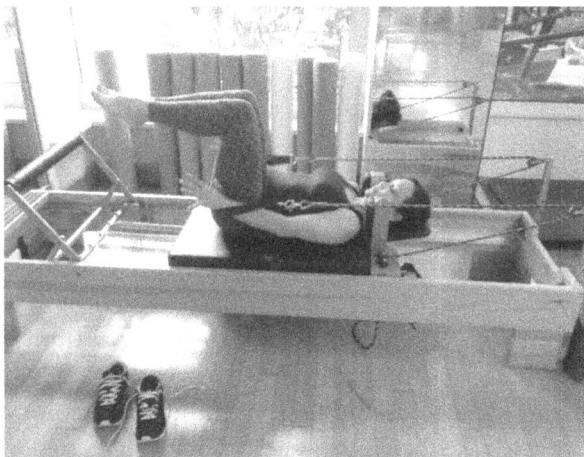

My wife Elena training on Pilates Reformer at the
Crown Plaza Hotel in Rome, Italy 2014

live in Manhattan. While in an elevator, a foreigner with a heavy ascent started asking me about supplements and workout tips.

We spent almost three weeks vacationing to celebrate our 25 wedding anniversary. We did not restrict our eating habits. By about the eighth day on vacation, I had gained 5 pounds and my body actually started telling me that this was happening because of all the eating I was doing. Consequently, I continued to eat the typical foods of the country we visited, but I cut down on the desserts. I also started eating healthy

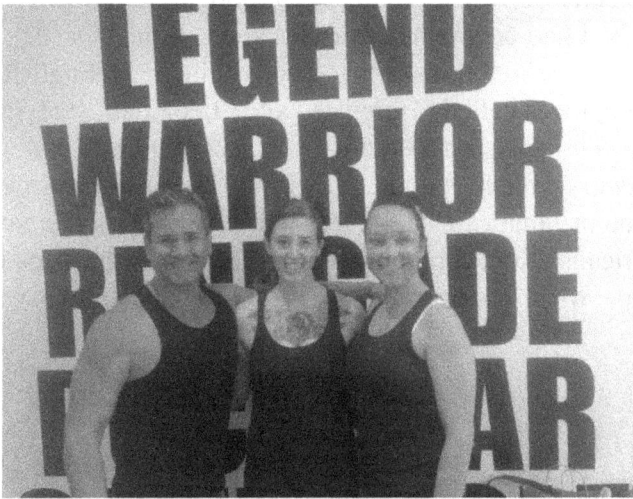

Training in NY City with our daughter-in-law, Kathryn Anta

breakfasts on the ship. Fortunately for us, Celebrity Cruises now have a healthy eating restaurant. By the time we got back to Miami, my weight had returned to normal. I think I even gained some muscle since my workout was heavy weight training and lots of walking to see the sites. At home, I usually train with weights, box, and practice Brazilian Jiu Jitsu. Then at night, I teach Krav Maga, Jeet Kune Do, Kung Fu and Muay Thai. I think that my body was recuperating more quickly since I was only doing weight training. As soon as I got back home, I continued the regular training and work routine which I love.

The Art of Breathing

The human body can survive without food for a few weeks and without water for just a few days, but it cannot survive without air for more than a few minutes. Joseph Pilates in his 1945 book, *"Return to Life through Contrology"* wrote: "Breathing is the first act of life and the last. Our very life depends on it. Lazy breathing converts the lungs into a cemetery for the deposition of disease, dying and dead germs as well as supplying an ideal haven for the multiplication of other harmful germs."

The art of breathing is an essential element in most physical art forms. In the Chinese martial arts (Kung fu, Tai Chi), it is called Chi (Qi). In India (Yoga), they call it Prana. In Japanese martial arts (Karate, Aikido), it is referred to as Ki. In Pilates, it is called diaphragm breathing. In my opinion, the best explanation comes from Angelo Sicilano, better known to us as "Charles Atlas," who won the title of "World's Most Perfectly Developed Man" in 1922. In his Dynamic Tension course he simply calls it deep lower breathing.

Never hold your breath while exercising. Holding your breath is dangerous; it could increase your blood pressure and tense your muscles.

It is said that there are 3 ways that a human being breaths.
1. High Chest
2. Chi Gong (like a baby)
3. Pilates

High chest is the way most of the population breaths, which is incorrect and unhealthy. Ask the average person to take a deep breath and their chest and shoulders will move. In all actuality, this is shallow breathing utilizing only three-fourths of your lungs.

The second way to breath is what the Japanese call Ki, what the Chinese call Chi, what the Indians call Prana, and is sometimes referred to as Yoga breathing.

Pilates breathing is diaphragmatic breathing similar to Yoga breathing.
Before beginning any Pilate's exercises, you should always begin by standing in anatomical pose and performing about eight breathing cycles of diaphragmatic breathing. During that pose, you will clear your mind of all outside thoughts and concentrate on making the mind-to-body connection.

In the West, we believe that the life center is the heart. In the East, it is believed that the tan tien (Chinese), hara (Japanese), a location just a few inches below the belly button is where life begins. The one point that both cultures can agree on is that oxygen is life! To acquire radiant health, fitness, and physical strength, you must relearn to breath. You must learn to breathe like a baby. If you witness a baby innocently sleeping in its cradle you will notice that the baby's chest does not move. You will see its belly, lower back and sides expanding as he/she inhales.

Diaphragm breathing furnishes the power to pump the blood through the heart. It oxygenates the blood and helps build new and stronger cells. It assists in carrying off waste products from the body. It will also utilize and exercise the entire lung area, as opposed to only using three-fourths of the lungs with shallow upper chest breathing. Correct breathing will also mobilize your spine and slow down the fusing that occurs with age.

If you look at any older physical culture course, you will notice that breathing fresh air outdoors was a staple of the program. In my Kung Fu system, Hung Gar, we have an advanced fifteen minute breathing and dynamic tension form called the Iron Wire. Okinawa and Japanese Goju Ryu Karate has a breathing tension form called Sanshin. Pilates, Yoga, and Tai Chi discipline also specialize in deep diaphragm breathing. Take one of these up for optimum health. Breathing exercises should be an essential part of your fitness program.

Martial Arts and other Activities

Martial arts is the staple of my success. I highly recommend everyone to train in a martial art. The belt system teaches you to set short term and long term goals. It teaches you self-discipline, respect, and self-defense. It gets you in shape and gives you flexibility to name a few of the many benefits.

Beware of the mystical traditional martial artist. I have heard it all. Things like, "My hands are registered with the FBI." "This is my board-breaking hand I have to be careful not to hurt you." "I can beat a UFC Fighter." "We have a killing blow. If I hit the bottom of your nose with the palm of my hand I will drive the bone through your brain and kill you." "If you attack me with a knife, I'll take it away from you without getting cut or stabbed." Believe me none of this is true.

Stay away from the cultish martial arts school. They tell you that they are the best system and the other martial arts are not as good. They tell you that if you leave the school you will never learn a high level of martial arts like theirs. The leader tries to convince you that he is the greatest martial artist that ever lived. In their extreme ego, they make their disciples do things like clean the school, and drop everything and run when they asks a disciple to do some errand like bringing them water. I once had an instructor that made his disciples cut his grass and do work around his house. Their disciples pay money to train, but this is what they get in exchange for real classes! Now, if someone is receiving training for free, then, of course, it could make sense that their tuition payment could include cleaning the school.

When looking for martial arts school, make sure that it is successful. If the school is not successful, how will they teach you to succeed? Make sure the instructors are fit and can perform the techniques. Would you go to a dentist with bad teeth? Ask yourself, "Are the instructors and students in this martial arts school being respectful to everyone in the class?"

I also strongly believe in strength training. Due to my back injury, I do my strength training at a gym. Yet, I believe in high intensity interval functional training. Many martial arts schools have great boot camps and kickboxing programs.
Beware of the franchise chains and affiliate programs. The national franchise chains can be purchased by anyone who has enough money to invest. The problem with this is that the trainers and owners are just following a program and may not have actual certification in specific martial arts and fitness. These franchises have a high turnaround of instructors and because of this, they will probably be hiring whomever is available whether they have specific experience or certification.

I know of a martial arts instructor in the greater Miami area that owned three national karate school chains and taught a national fitness kickboxing affiliate. He was a kung fu instructor that called himself a master, yet no one knows who promoted him to the rank of Master, and no one has ever seen him perform. His schools are run by teenagers and his fitness kickboxing programs are run by personal trainers and karate practitioners. When he opened the franchise he started teaching karate forms that originated from Tae Kwon Do. He eventually left this national karate franchise. When he closed one of the three schools, he opened a new location that only teaches this fitness type of kickboxing with which he is affiliated. Currently, he is recruiting physical education teachers to teach kickboxing. None of his instructors have spent the years it takes to be proficient in kickboxing.

Not all affiliate programs are bad. The instructor teaching the course is what determines whether the program is good or bad.

Chapter 3

Health and Nutrition

Sanitas Per Escam
Health Through Food

Six Vital Nutrients

Nutrients will provide energy and muscle development, and will keep you disease free. Kid's today eat fast foods, junk food, and have diets high in calories and fats. This is why kids today are having health problems that were once only seen in adults. Poor eating habits are linked to obesity, heart disease and diabetes. Your body needs the following six nutrients: protein, carbohydrates, fats, vitamins, minerals, and water. We must include all six nutrients in our diet to stay young, healthy, and alive.

Protein: You need plenty of protein for growth and for post-exercise tissue building. As we age, we lose muscle mass. We need to feed our muscles with protein for muscle growth. Protein is needed for nourishing, maintaining, and replacing muscles, organs, bones, enzymes, hormone, immune system, and cell membranes. Stay away from soy protein which increases your estrogen levels.

Carbohydrates: Carbohydrates are your body fuel. They are your primary source of energy. The brain, nervous systems, and blood cells strongly rely on carbohydrates. Low and zero carbohydrate diets are very dangerous for a growing child.

Fats: Fats are the body's main energy source and protects your internal organs. There are several types of fats. Some are good and essential and some are bad for you. There are saturated, monounsaturated fats. You should restrict the intake of saturated fats like whole milk, hamburgers and lunch meats. Choose to consume olive oil and fish which are high in monounsaturated fats.

Vitamins: Vitamins are substances that are present in foods when those foods are prepared as close to the way God made them as possible. The more processed the food is, the less vitamins you'll find. For your child to develop their body and grow up healthy they need a variety of vitamins. To stay healthy and fit as we age, vitamin and mineral supplement are recommended since most people do not eat the right nutrients to supply the proper amount of vitamins. A vitamin and mineral supplement should supplement our healthy eating habits. It should not replace healthy eating even though today's foods do not carry the same nutrients that they did 50 years ago.

Minerals: Just like vitamins minerals are also present in our foods and we must ensure that we get the right portions in order to stay strong, fit, and healthy. Minerals are inorganic substances found in rocks and in the soil that enter into our diet through plants and through the animals that eat plants. Since our soil is lacking minerals today, our foods are also lacking minerals. This is why we need to supplement our diet with certain mineral supplements.

Water: Last, but not least, is water. Drinking pure water is of the utmost importance in order to live a healthy life and even to lose weight. Approximately one-half to one ounce of water per pound of body weight is recommended for children and adults on a daily basis. When exercising in the summer, you should be drinking even higher quantities of water. You should hydrate before, during, and after exercise and play. Your body is approximately 70% water. Sadly, 75% of Americans are chronically dehydrated. Don't wait until you are thirsty to drink water. In 37% of Americans, the thirst mechanism is so weak that it is often mistaken for hunger. Drinking water throughout the day will increase your energy levels. Water will also help remove toxins from your body and fight off the common cold.

Make sure that you drink lots of purified water on a daily basis. Tap water has numerous environmental toxins, such as chlorine, pesticides, parasites, and chemicals from perfumes, caffeine, and numerous other things dumped into it. While you should space your water consumption evenly throughout the day the best time to drink water is when you first wake up in the morning. Drink water before breakfast since your body needs hydration from all the hours in which you were sleeping.

Water is great for you. It will help you burn fat, suppress hunger, and replenish your skin, making it look youthful again.

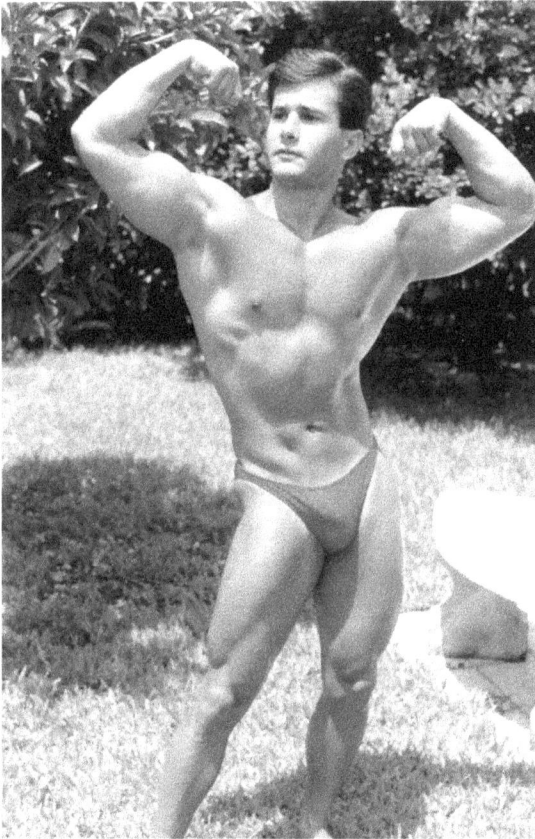

In 1985 at 28 years old

Vitamins and Minerals in your Food

Today's fruits, vegetables, and herbs do not have the vitamins and minerals that they did when your grandparents were kids. According to the USDA the vitamin and mineral content of our foods has drastically gone down in the last 30 years. In 1936, a group of Doctors brought to the US Senate a warning that the mineral content in the soil was eroding which was causing the fruits and vegetables to lose their nutritional content. In the 1939, Jethro Koss wrote a book entitled, "Back to Eden." Koss warned of the depletion of nutrients in our soil. There are numerous reasons why fruits and vegetables have lost their vitamins and minerals. The main reasons for soil depletion are the use of pesticides, chemicals fertilizers, genetic modifications, and the developing of hybrid crops.

Some nutritionists believe that today it takes ten servings of vegetables to equal what could previously be found in just one serving fifty years ago. Below is the loss of vitamin and minerals in our fruits since 1975:
- Apples – 41% decrease in Vitamin A
- Sweet Peppers – 31% decrease in Vitamin C
- Watercress – 88% decrease in Iron
- Broccoli – 50% decrease in Calcium and Vitamin A
- Cauliflower – 45% decrease in Vitamin C, 48% in Vitamin B1, and 47% in Vitamin B2
- Collards Greens – 45% decrease in Vitamin A and 85% in Magnesium

The best way to get all the vitamin, minerals and anti-oxidants from your fruits and vegetables is to buy them organic. Farmers' Markets are great for fresh, organic, seasonal fruits, herbs and vegetables. It is still better to eat fruits that are not organic then junk food and sugar filled desserts.

To stay young eat fruits and vegetables on a daily basis. If you don't like vegetables, then put them a natural smoothie and/or get a juicer and juice your fruits and vegetables. My breakfast is a fruit, vegetable, and herb smoothie.

Even though I live in Doral, a suburb of Miami with a paved backyard, I have made my own organic garden. I love waking up and picking herbs for my morning smoothie. This assures

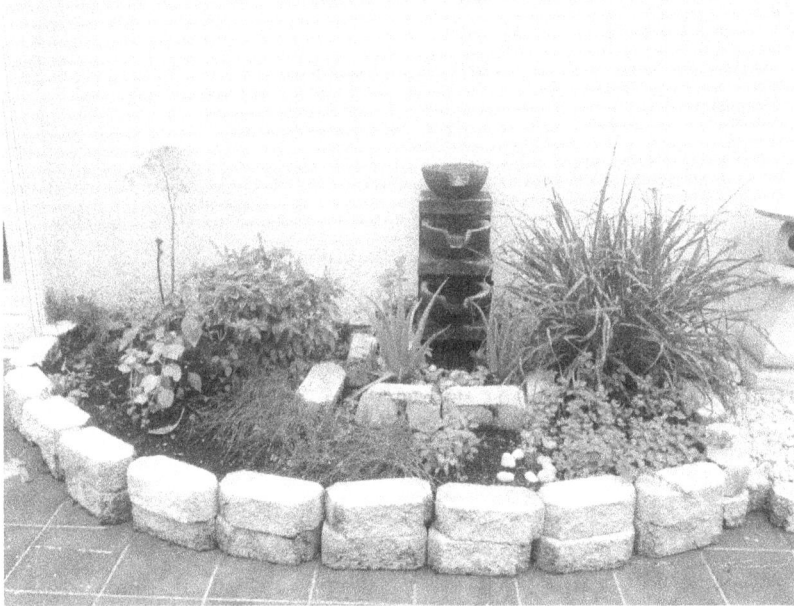

My backyard organic garden

me that it is truly organic. I also have tomatoes in my garden. I have never like tomatoes until my first home harvest. Home-grown tomatoes taste great and are incredibly juicy. When tomatoes are in season, it is great to pick them right before your lunch or dinner.

Getting Started on a Healthy Nutrition Program

"Let food be thy medicine and medicine be thy food" - Hippocrates.

You've heard the old saying "You are what you eat," right? 80% of your success in a fitness program comes from a healthy nutrition program. Success will come when you combine healthy eating, food supplements, and a safe and effective fitness training program. It is important to avoid injuries for longevity's sake.

I don't believe in dieting. I believe in healthy eating. In this book you will see a section on Good Foods, Bad Foods, Eating Five to Six Small Meals a Day, Eating One Serving from the Protein Section in Each Meal, and One Serving from the Carbohydrates or Vegetable Sections. Following the Good Food selection and avoiding the Bad Foods will help you loss fat. Eating more from the vegetable section and less from the carbohydrates section will be more beneficial and help you loss fat faster and keep you healthier.

In a nutshell you can eat lean red meat, and all the poultry, and fish that you like with a carbohydrate. Organic meats are preferable. As for carbohydrates, eat all the vegetables you like. You can substitute full meals for smoothies with protein. Also, you can substitute some meals for protein drinks or protein bars.

If you are eating healthy six days a week, you can afford to break your healthy eating habits once a week. You can take off one day as a "cheat day" where you eat pizza, hamburger, fries, cake, cookies, ice cream or whatever you have an urge for. This method will actually help you, since you've been restricting your calories, your body feels that it is starving. When you have a cheat day with higher calories your body goes back to regular mode.

Another important point is not to use soy protein. Soy brings up your estrogen level. I personally only eat red meat once a month. I also have not drunk a soda in over twelve years. You should have a log to write down your statistics, goals, exercise program, and the foods you eat. People that write down their goals and keep track of what they are eating have a higher rate of success.

We cannot prescribe diets or supplements, so these are merely suggestions of what has worked for us. Consult with your doctor before starting any diet, taking supplements or beginning an exercise program.

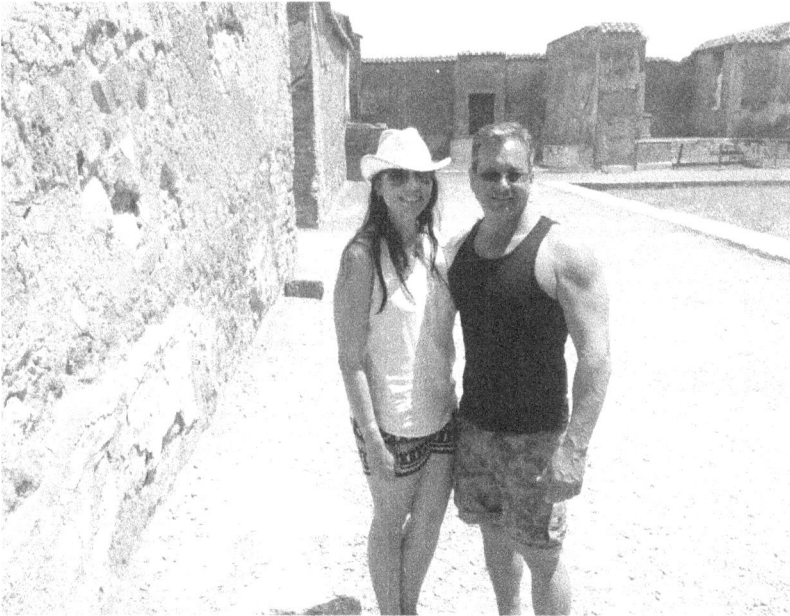

Celebrating our 25 year wedding anniversary in Pompeii, Italy 2014

There are many types of healthy and unhealthy foods. The list below is just some suggested ideas.

Healthy Food List

Proteins	Carbohydrates Fruits	Vegetables
Chicken	Brown Rice	Carrots
Turkey	Whole Wheat Pasta	Garlic
Ground Turkey	Whole Wheat Bread	Spinach
Tuna	Potato	Lettuce
All Fish	Sweet Potato	Onions
Lean Meats	Yogurt	Black Olives
Eggs	All Fruits	Green Peppers
Peanut Butter	Pumpkin	Celery
Nuts	Corn	Green Beans
Veal	Whole Wheat Bagel	Peas
Vegi Burgers	Beans	Brussels Sprouts
Low Fat Milk	Quinoa	Asparagus
Sashimi	Sushi (protein, carbohydrate, fat)	All Vegetables

Unhealthy Food List

Proteins	Carbohydrates	Others
Pork	Cakes	Mayonnaise
Ham	Ice Cream	Syrups
Hot Dogs	Cookies	Margarine
Prime Ribs	Fried Rice	Sour Cream
Hamburgers	French Fries	Cheese Sauces
Salami	Marshmallows	Fatty Dressings
Bologna	Potato Chips	Sodas
Corned Beef	Egg Rolls	Diet Soda
Bacon	Candy	Salt
Fatty Meats	White Flour/Sugar	Sugar Substitutes

This is just partial list of healthy and unhealthy foods. Eat foods as close to the way God made them. Use organic food when possible. Drink lots of water. Use sea salt to season your food if needed. Only fry in coconut oil. Do not drink sodas, alcohol, or beer. Stay away from cigarettes and drugs. Do not microwave your food. Eat 5 to 6 small meals a day. For more information on fitness and healthy eating go to our blog:

MartialArtsAndFitness.typepad.com

Herbs/Supplements/Juice

Below, I am writing about the herbs and supplements that I am currently using. I change my supplements at times.

Life Extension Brand

• Extraordinary Enzymes for digestion.

• L-Argine for circulation and Human Growth Hormone

•Vitamin C and Super Omega 3 for your heart health

• Antaxanthin raises testosterone levels

•Melatonin to help sleep and increase HGH (Human Growth Hormone)

• Natural Prostate

•Vitamin D3 since most people are vitamin D deficient

• CoQ10 for heart health

• Resveratrol for the heart

• Brain Shield

• Pomi-T for the prostate

• Milk Thistle for the liver

• Magnesium to prevent crams and muscle spasm

• Super Miraforte to raise testosterone

•GH Pituitary Support Night Formula to raise HGH (Human Growth Hormone)

Himalaya Brand

• Garcinia to suppress appetite

• Turmeric for pain relief and anti-inflammatory

• Ashwagandha raises testosterone levels

I also take whey protein to supplement my protein intake and fenugreek to raise testosterone and HGH (human growth hormone).

Five out of seven days a week (unless I'm in a hurry after my mobility exercises) I make my morning juice. First I'll go outside to my small, suburban, organic garden. I pick some moringa leaves, mint, lemongrass, sage, basil, Mexican Tarragon, and cilantro. I then add cinnamon, maca, flaxseed, turmeric, pumpkin seed, and ginger. Next, I mix it with either cantaloupe, watermelon, bananas, strawberries, mangos or organic mixed berries. I will also add protein.

What is Moringa?

Moringa Oleifera is also known as the Miracle Tree and the Tree of Life. It is originally from the Himalayans, yet today it is cultivated throughout the world, South America, Africa, the Caribbean and even here in Florida. Today, moringa is also being harvested in different countries in the continent of Africa to help fight malnutrition.

When you hear of all the many benefits of the moringa tree, it might sound like a sales pitch by the old west charlatan, snake-oil salesmen because it truly sounds like magic. Scientists call moringa the most nutrient rich plant ever studied.

Moringa leaves have been used in traditional medicine passed down for centuries in many cultures. In the ancient Indian tradition of Ayurveda, they use the leaves of the moringa tree prevent 300 diseases. Today's modern scientific community has done more than 750 studies, articles and other publications that have included moringa.

In order to live fit and healthy at 57 years old, I eat healthy, workout hard doing martial arts and strength training, doing joint mobility, and I also take numerous nutritional supplements. Yet, my favorite supplement is moringa. I planted five moringa trees in my backyard. The first one was planted almost three months ago. I dry my moringa leaves and mix it with other fruits and herbs in my morning drink. If I'm in hurry or traveling, I take moringa capsules from a company called, King Moringa. I know that most people will not take the time to grow organic Moringa trees, pick the leaves, and dry them before ingesting them, so I highly recommend moringa capsules. Since I started taking moringa, I have not caught a cold. I start feeling a sore throat, but it doesn't progress with other symptoms and it goes away quickly. Before I began taking moringa I was always getting sick.

Moringa is rich in Vitamin A, Vitamin B1, Vitamin B2, Vitamin B3, Vitamin C, Calcium, Chromium, Copper, Iron, Magnesium, Manganese, Phosphorus, Potassium, all essential amino acids (Protein,) and Zinc. Moringa leaves have seven times the Vitamin C of oranges, four times the Vitamin A of carrots, four times the calcium of milk, three times the potassium of bananas and two times the protein of yogurt. Those with good health find that moringa boosts their energy and sustained well-being. The greatest benefits have been seen with people who have average or poor health. Below are some of the known benefits of moringa.

Anti-Cholesterol
Helps control diabetes
Gives a feeling of general wellness
Nourishes that body's immune system
Great for circulation
Regulates blood pressure
Increases the natural defenses of the body
Helps with mental clarity
Nourishes the eyes and the brain
Detoxifies your body
Can help you loss weight
Promotes healthy digestion
Great antioxidant
High alkalinity helps balance your body's pH level
Anti-aging benefits
Increases Libido
Anti-inflammatory
Helps your body recovery from workouts
Will help you sleep better
Keeps your skin healthy
Promotes healthy liver and the kidney

To get optimal results with moringa, use it steadily for at least three months. One bottle will last you a month. I use and recommend the brand called King Moringa.

Garcinia Cambogia for Weight Control

Garcinia Cambogia is the best supplement I've ever tried to for the purpose of burning fat. It is also the only supplement I've ever taken that suppresses my appetite. Garcinia is able to burn fat and even stop fat from ever forming. It also gives you energy and stops carbohydrate cravings.

The fat-burning secret of Garcinia Cambogia is that the fruit contains a large amount of Hydroxycitric Acid (HCA), which is the active ingredient that aids weight loss. The way it works as an appetite suppressant is that it increases the amount of serotonin in your body. That means that you'll be feeling happier and more content. Garcinia tells your brain when to feel fuller and stop eating.

HCA is the main ingredient found in Garcinia, so when choosing a supplement, make sure that it has at least 60% HCA. It is also important to make sure that it is pure Garcinia Cambodia and has no other ingredients such as vitamins, minerals, or herbs. I've tried Garcinia along with other herbs and minerals and it did not work as effectively. Pure Garcinia Cambogia also costs less.

Take one pure Garcinia tablet without any other supplement on an empty stomach twice a day 15-30 minutes before a meal. I use Himalayan brand of Garcinia. When I first started taking this supplement, the bottle said to take it after your meals. It did work, but I got much better results and appetite suppression when I began taking it 15-30 minutes before a meal.

Hygiene

Hygiene is very important for our health, but stay away from commercial products that are full of harmful chemicals. My shampoo, shaving cream, tooth paste, deodorant, and soap are all natural and organic.

Last year, I was asked on Facebook to explain what creams I used to stay younger looking. I was surprised to hear that question, since I've never used any creams. I even break the anti-wrinkle rules by sun bathing without using sunscreen. I'm not recommending for others to do this. I've been sunbathing since I was around 9 years old when my parents had to move from New York to Miami Beach due to my illness and allergic condition to cold weather. From the age of 19 unto the age of 29, during my bodybuilding days, I would spend the weekend at the beach.

Ever since I was just a young kid, I have read in a muscle magazine how soap dries up the natural oils of your skin. For this reason, I only wash my face with soap whenever I shower. Until a month ago I washed my face with a natural organic soap. Due to my wife's persuasion, I started using a natural organic face scrub instead of soap.

I use a natural and organic fluoride-free toothpaste. I never let the dentist use fluoride when getting my teeth cleaned. Fluoride is a highly toxic substance. It can cause brain damage, arthritic symptoms, bone fractures, and thyroid gland issues.

How to Increase Testosterone

Testosterone is a hormone produced by both men and women. Men have higher testosterone levels than women. It plays a role in puberty and fertility. It also affects sexual desire. During puberty a boy's testosterone level increases and he starts to become a man. During puberty, his voice begins to change, his shoulder begin to widen, he becomes more muscular, his facial features become more masculine, and he begins to grow hair on his face and legs. Before puberty 10- to 11-year-old boys have testosterone levels which could range from 7-130 ng/dl. As boys enter puberty at around the ages of 12 and 13, this level could increase to 800 ng/dl. Between the ages of 14 and 18, these levels can increase even further to as high as 1200 ng/dl. An adult male in his twenties will average between 270-1,070 ng/hl. To feel healthy and strong, testosterone levels must be maintained at higher levels.

Unfortunately, testosterone levels in most men begin to decline as they reach their 30's. The Mayo clinic did a study that claims that each year after the age of 30, a man's testosterone level drops around one percent. Over thirteen million men have lower-than-normal testosterone levels. This could mean a decrease in their sex life, and a loss in power, confidence, and the ability to succeed in life. Low testosterone could also bring physical and emotional changes known as andropause.

Fast foods and lack of exercise contributes to lowering your testosterone levels. Low testosterone and high estrogen will leave you weak, fat, and at a much higher risk for cancer, diabetes, and heart disease.

An optimal testosterone level increases sexual potency, inhibits wrinkling, and improves skin texture and elasticity. It improves immunity and healing. It reduces body fat, and increases strength, energy and lean muscle. It will increase mental functioning, emotional stability, improve cardiovascular endurance and it even improves hair texture and thickness.

Low testosterone and high estrogen is why we have such small amounts of real men, also known as Alpha Males. An Alpha Male is a strong take-charge warrior, hunter, and protector of his family. He is also a risk taker.

I believe that we are going through a crisis in our country which is called the "Feminization of America" where men are becoming, as Arnold Schwarzenegger puts it, "Girlie Men." This is the exact opposite of the Alpha Male. Part of the feminization of America is due to low testosterone and high estrogen.

Testosterone can be increased by heavy, low-repetition strength training, and high-intensity, interval, cardio training instead of long distance jogging. Nutrition, numerous kinds of herbs and bio-identical hormones are also beneficial.

To increase testosterone, you must live a healthy life. Alcohol, some prescription drugs, and recreational drugs lower your testosterone levels.

Marijuana lowers your testosterone and raises your estrogen levels. A characteristic of high marijuana uses in men is gynecomastia. Gynecomastia is also known as bitch tits in the bodybuilding world and man boobs to the general public. Gynecomastia is caused by a hormone imbalance. When the ratio between testosterone and estrogen tips in favor of estrogen, the body responds by creating excessive breast tissue. Animal studies have shown that exposure to marijuana can result in a decrease in testosterone levels, a reduction of testicular size, and abnormalities in the form and function of sperm. The testosterone levels decrease and estrogen stays the same.

Go to the herb/supplement page to read about the supplements I use to bring up my testosterone.

How to Increase HGH (Human Growth Hormone)

As you grow older, the Human Growth Hormone (HGH or GH) decreases. Human Growth Hormone is also known as somatotropin or somatropin. It is a peptide hormone that stimulates growth, cell reproduction, and regeneration in humans and other animals.

HGH deficiency begins for most people in their 20's. This, in turn, leads to a reduction in lean body mass, reduction in bone mineral density, and an increase in body fat especially in the abdominals. You begin to look and feel older as HGH declines.

HGH gives you energy. It keeps you looking young, muscular, with vitality and strength. HGH is a hormone produced by the pituitary gland. The human growth hormone builds and strengthens muscles and bones. We produce the most HGH during adolescence.

To increase your HGH, you must do short, heavy, strength training. Never workout for longer than an hour. I've been known to do heavy 30 to 45 min strength training workouts.

There are also some supplements which can help increase HGH in conjunction with strength training. Here is a list of some of the supplements I take or have taken to increase my HGH:

• L-Argine
• L-Lysine
• Fenugreek
• Moringa
• Vitamin D
• Liquid Melatonin
• Life Extension GH Pituitary Support Night Formula

Chapter 4
Ageless Warriors

Caleb, An Ageless Warrior

"Now then, just as the Lord promised, he has kept me alive for forty-five years since the time he said this to Moses, while Israel moved about in the wilderness. So here I am today, eighty-five years old! I am still as strong today as the day Moses sent me out; I'm just as vigorous to go out to battle now as I was then" (Joshua 14:10-11 NIV).

What do Centenarians have in Common?

We cannot defy time, yet we can slow down the aging process with proper eating habits, healthy living, and by staying active through training. National Geographic Magazine November 2005 issue featured this article: *"The Secrets of Living Longer"* which focuses on specific people groups where centenarians (people who live to be 100 years old) are frequent.

In that article, the three diverse groups of centurions interviewed were the Seven Day Adventists from the United States; the Sardinians (inhabitants on an island in Italy); and the people from Okinawa (an island which is now part of Japan). Interestingly, they have discovered similarities between these people groups. They all ate different healthy diets and had different religions yet what they had in common was that they work physically hard, yet relaxed and had calm minds. Even though their religions were different, they all believed in a higher deity and ate healthy fresh foods. There were also some key habits which they held in common. They don't smoke. They put their family first. They are active every day. They keep socially engaged. Their diets consist of fruits, vegetables, and whole grains.

The National Institute on Aging says that 70 percent of longevity is determined by your lifestyle and only 30 percent of longevity determined by your genes. The Bible also clearly speaks against gluttony in Proverbs 23:21 by telling us that drunkards and gluttons will become poor. I truly believe that if we follow the advice given in the Bible, there would be a very little obese or unhealthy people. For that matter, if we follow the eating advice of most religions there wouldn't be a need for this book.

The Japanese believe that everyone has a reason for being. They believe that this is what makes life worth living. Living or searching for your purpose is the key to longevity. I have heard of numerous stories of someone passing away right after retiring. This could be because their job provided a purpose for living. Having purpose could be one of the secrets that most centenarians share.

There are approximately 125,000 centenarians in the United States as per the U.S. Census. They estimate that there could be one million centenarians in America and six million centenarians worldwide by the year 2050. The Bible says, "Then

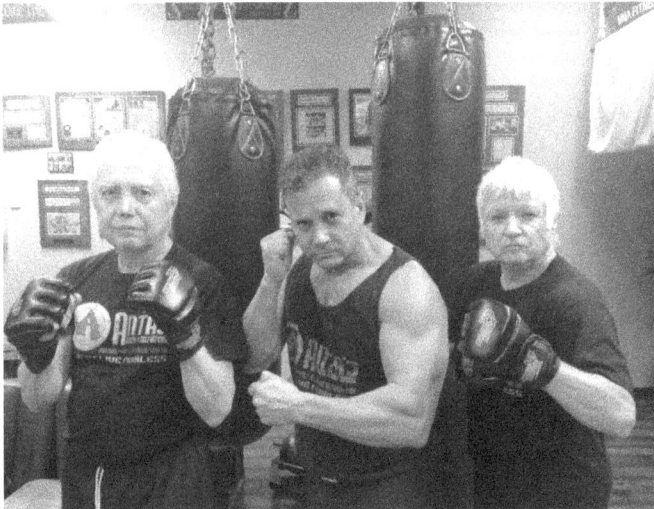

You are never too old to start. With Krav Maga students Victor Suarez 71 and Linda Dillard 69

the Lord said, 'My Spirit shall not abide in man forever, for he is flesh: his days shall be 120 years'" (Genesis 6:3, NIV) God's plan was for us to live to be 120, yet very few people live to be 90.

When animals in the wild eat their natural diet, they will live an average of ten times the number of years it takes them to reach maturity. A human lifespan is less than five times the number of years it takes to reach maturity. That means that animals live double the amount of years of humans.

Famous Ageless Warriors

Jack LaLanne (September 26, 1914 - January 23, 2011) and
Helio Gracie (October 1, 1913 – January 29, 2009) are two
men that I admire. I would love to have met them, but
unfortunately, I was never had that opportunity. Both Jack and
Helio lived into their nineties and kept on training until their
death. Jack was a fitness guru, inventor and broke many fitness
records. Helio changed the
martial arts world by taking
challenge matches and
beating other martial artist
with his improved version of
Jiu Jitsu known as Gracie Jiu
Jitsu. His eldest son, Rorian,
developed the UFC
(Ultimate Fighting
Championship) and his son,
Royce, won the first UFC.

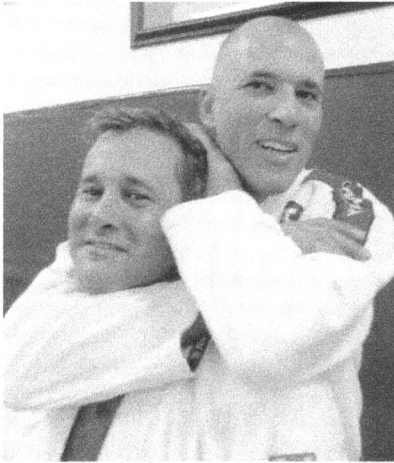

Training with Royce Gracie age 47, 2013

Today all UFC fighters train in Gracie Jiu Jitsu.
There were many similarities between these two great men.
They both ate healthy, exercised until their death, did not drink,
smoke, or did drugs. They both changed the world for the
better.

In this section you will read about these two famous Ageless
Warriors and some other Ageless Warriors that I admire.

Jack LaLanne

Jack LaLanne lived to be 96 years old. He was a fitness, exercise, and nutritional expert. Jack had the first-ever fitness show on TV which ran nationally for over 34 years. He invented numerous exercise machines and was a motivational speaker who is has been called "the godfather of fitness" "The King of Fitness" and the "First Fitness Superhero." He was an innovator and a man ahead of his time because he was leading the fitness world before fitness was cool. He was a very patriotic man that loved this great nation.

You might remember him for the Jack LaLanne Power Juicer infomercial. Jack had been juicing since his teens. Lalane also developed the first pin-weighted exercise machine. He developed the first cabled, pulley and leg extension machine. Most of you have done jumping jacks, right? Well, why do you think they are called "Jumping Jacks"?

As a child, Jack was a weak, sickly kid addicted to sugar. At age 15, he went with his mother to a Paul Bragg health and nutrition seminar. This changed his life. From that moment forward, Jack was motivated to focus on his diet and exercise.

Some of Jack's quotes are, "Life is great when you're in shape." "Health is wealth." "It's a lifestyle. It's something you do the rest of your life. How long are you going to keep breathing? How long do you keep eating? You just do it." "The only way you get that fat off is to eat less and exercise more."

Every year on his birthday Jack would do an amazing feat or break a personal record. When he turned 43 in 1957, he performed more than 1,000 push-ups in 23 minutes on the *"You Asked For It"* television show. At the age of 60, Jack swam from Alcatraz Island to Fisherman's Wharf in San Francisco while handcuffed, shackled and towing a boat.

Today Jack's wife, Elaine LaLanne, who is 88 and had been married to Jack for 59 years, continues the family fitness legacy as a health and fitness speaker. Jack was quoted to say, "If you are around her for any length of time, you will find her enthusiasm for life is contagious. She can do push-ups and chin-ups. She's a terrific golfer, expert water skier, and swimmer. She's a lecturer, author, civic leader, and business woman. In fact, she runs BeFit Enterprises. She's a super wife and a good friend. To me she is living proof of all that a woman can be!"

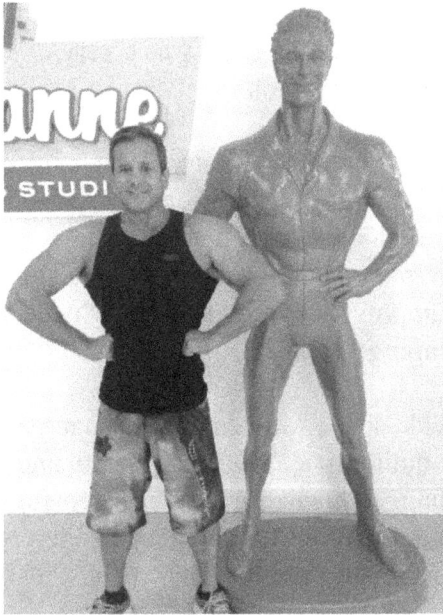

As a kid in New York, I loved watching Jack on TV and dreaming of looking like him when I grew up. Outside of the Steve Reeves Hercules reruns, you would never see a bodybuilder on TV. As an adult, I read Jack's book and was inspired

Jack LaLanne Health Studio in Orlando 2014

by him to workout hard and set goals as I aged. I was more impressed by Jack when he was in his 90's than I was when he was a fit, muscular 20 years old. For more information on Jack LaLanne and his products, log on to his website: www.JackLaLanne.com

Helio Gracie

Helio Gracie, together with his brother Carlos, changed the world with their development of a martial arts system called Gracie Jiu Jitsu. Helio was born in Brazil on October 1, 1913, and passed away on January 29, 2009. He taught and grappled until his death at 95. Carlos also lived a long and fit life, living to the age of 92.

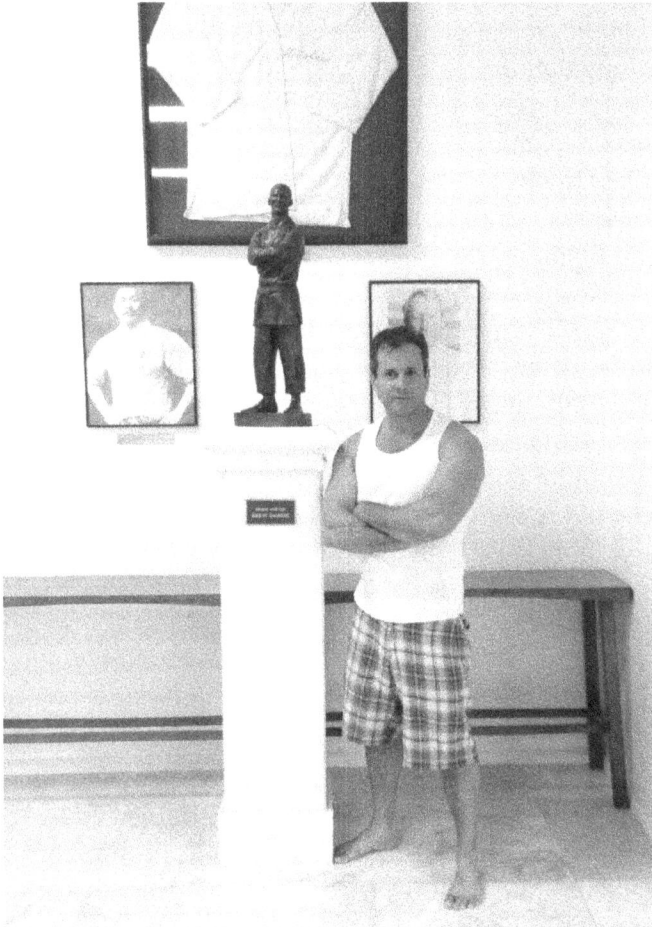

By the Helio Gracie Statue at Valente Brothers Jiu Jitsu 2013

Helio is known as the most important figure in Brazilian Jiu Jitsu and, along with his son, was instrumental in changing the martial arts world. His son, Rorian, developed the UFC (Ultimate Fighting Championship) and his other son, Royce, was the first UFC champion.

Helio followed a special diet developed by his brother, Carlos. It was a diet of food combining that they called the "Gracie Diet." He did not drink, smoke, take drugs or eat junk food. Helio's children and grandchildren also continue to follow these eating habits.

Helio was 5'9"and 139 pounds. He took many challenges to prove that Gracie Jiu Jitsu was the best and complete fighting system. He was Brazil's number one ranked fighter in Vale-Tudo (no-holds-barred) for most of his competitive career.

I train in Gracie Jiu Jitsu at Valente Brothers Jiu Jitsu under instructors, Jimmy Robertson and Burak Eyilik, who both trained directly under Helio. Jimmy knew Helio very well. He once told me that he would go out to eat with Helio and that Helio would look at people in their sixties and seventies and say, "I would never want to look like them." That was when Helio was in his nineties! I also had the privilege to train with Helio's son and first UFC (Ultimate Fighting Championship, Royce Gracie.

The Valente Brothers grandfather, Syllo, and father, Pedro Valente Sr., both trained in Jiu Jitsu under Helio. Pedro Valente Sr. holds the highest rank achievable in Jiu Jitsu, the 10th degree red belt. All three Valente Brothers trained and were promoted to black belt under Helio. The Valenti brothers have pledge to continue Helio's legacy by training and teaching Jiu Jitsu just like Helio did.

Bobby Cruz

Christian Pastor/Salsa Singer

Bobby Cruz is 77 years old, yet he actually looks 20 years younger. He was born on February 2, 1937. He is a Puerto Rican born salsa singer, Christian pastor, minister, and the apostle of Iglesia Casa de Alabanza. He is best known for his success beginning in 1965 as part of the duo, **Richie Ray & Bobby Cruz**. Richie Ray and Bobby Cruz won a total of nine gold record awards.

Today, he is as popular as ever selling, out stadiums in Puerto Rico, Columbia, and other parts of the world. Most 77-year-olds are retired, reminiscing of their past, but not Bobby! He continues touring. Bobby has to stay in shape to be able to tour and sing throughout the world at age 77.

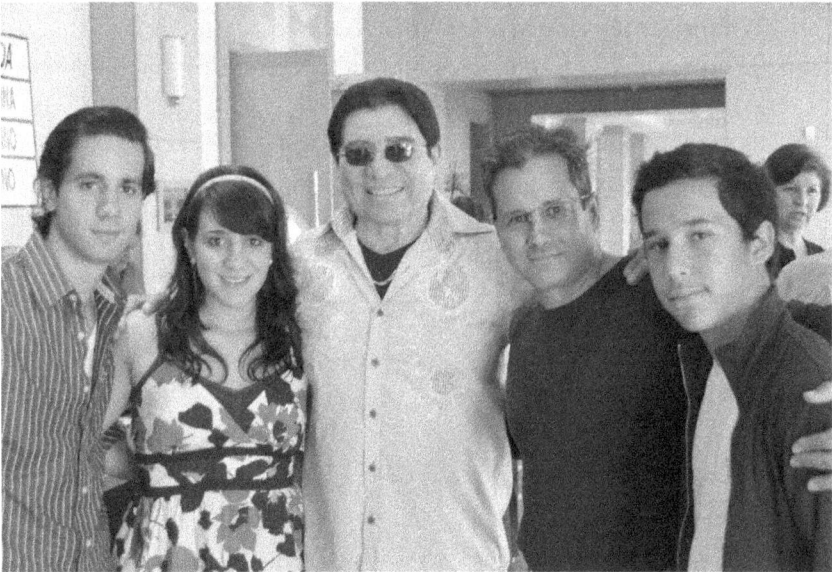

From left to right: Julio's nephew and niece, David Josiah and Abigail Slentz, Bobby Cruz at age 73, Julio, and Julio's son, Jon-Paul

I know Bobby as a friend and spiritual leader. As of today, I have never met a pastor with the Biblical knowledge of Apostle Cruz. I was baptized, married, and presented my first son to the Lord in Iglesia Casa de Alabanza when he was the head Pastor. I spend about five years attending his church. I left Iglesia Casa de Alabanza, for a period of twenty years, during which time I attended two different churches. Four years ago, I returned to Iglesia Casa de Alabanza. Now it is pastored by his son and one of my best friends, Bobby Cruz, Jr., Bobby Jr. is 50 years old and looks as if he was in his late 30's. Bobby Jr. works out in the gym and jogs.

I'll never forget back in the late 1980's when my father told me how much he admired Bobby because he was a man's man. Even though he was a pastor, he was a powerful and tough guy that showed presence and high self-esteem. My dad would praise the way Bobby walked, talked and carried himself..

Whenever he sees me, he bows to me, calls me Sensei (teacher in Japanese), and usually tells me how great I look. This is a great compliment since Bobby himself has always kept himself in great shape by working out. This last Sunday, I looked at Bobby and the thought came to my mind: "Bobby looks better today than when he was younger." So, I went to him and told him that he looks better with age. He is truly an Ageless Warrior.

Jhoon Rhee

Jhoon Rhee is known as the father of American Tae Kwon Do, the creator of the karate safety equipment and musical forms. He is 82 years old and was born on January 7, 1932. He was a training partner with Bruce Lee. He even did a few kung fu movies. Rhee's motto is, "One hundred years of wisdom in a 21-year old body." In his 60's and 70's he would drop before starting a seminar and do 100 easy pushups. His flexibility is remarkable doing full splits and holding his leg over his head while giving a lecture. He arrived in America in the 1950s and

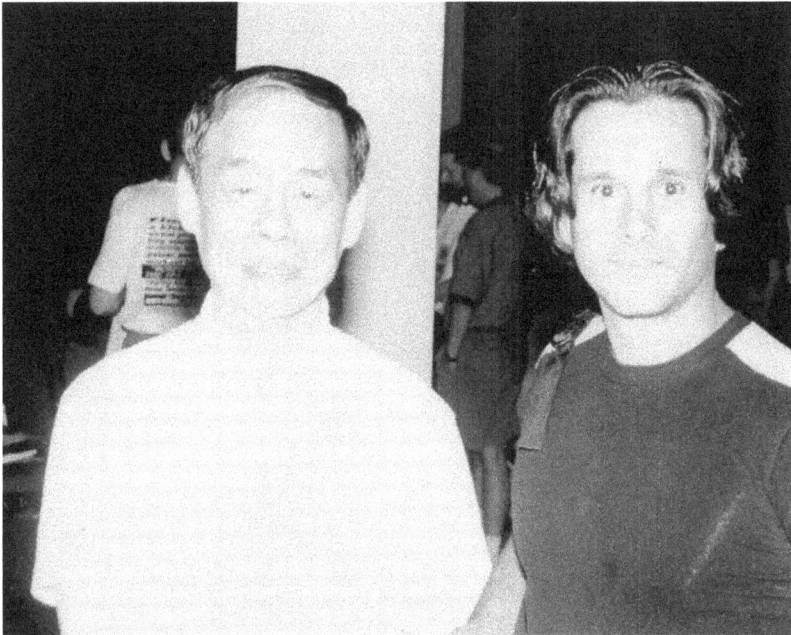

With Jhoon Rhee in 1999. Rhee was 67 and Anta was 44

began spreading his martial arts philosophy in America and around the world. He is one of the world's most famous and influential martial artists. He loves America, his adopted country, and is a great American patriot.

In 1965, he started Rhee's U.S. Congressional Tae Kwon Do Club. One of the first students was Vice President Joe Biden. More than 350 members of Congress have attended Rhee's classes. Nineteen members of Congress have earned black belts under him.

I have met and spoken to Jhoon Rhee a few times. I was a speaker at the NAPMA World Martial Arts conference as well as Master Rhee. We were sitting at a table having lunch when one of his students that was sitting at the table had heard that I was in my forties and told Rhee. Rhee's reply to me was "People like you in Miami and I in Washington D.C. are going to change the world by staying fit and looking young." Wow, I felt as if I were on top of the world getting complimented by this legend in the martial arts.

Sig (Sigmund) Klien

Sig Klien was born in Germany on April 10, 1902, and died on May 24, 1987. He lived to be 85 years old. Sig operated his famous New York City studio, Sigmund Klein Gymnasium, located at 717 Seventh Avenue, New York City.

Sig began bodybuilding at 15 years old. He married Prof. Louis Atilla's youngest daughter and took over running Atilla's gym in 1927. Atilla was a professional strongman. I was lucky

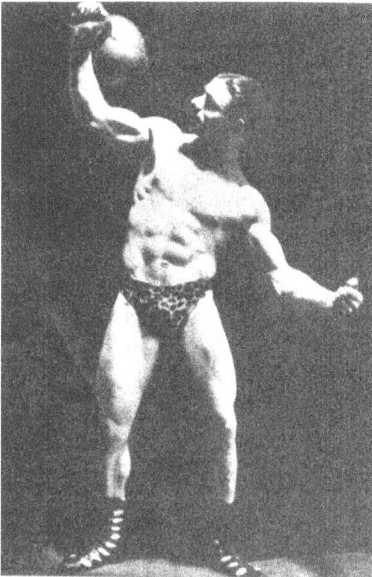 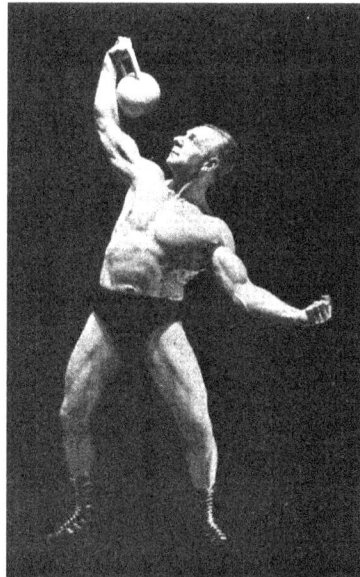

Age 22 in 1924   *Age 57 in 1959*

enough to meet someone that had trained in Klein's Gym. I also met Frank Adler, a Masters Boxer, who was in his 70's around two years ago. He is an interesting man who trained and was a sparring partner with Joe Frazier before Frazier became the world's heavy boxing champion. Frank was interested in learning how to use Indian clubs to heal and strengthen his shoulders to enhance his boxing for longevity. He asked me if I knew who Sig Klien was. My answer was sure I do. He was a

149

strongman and bodybuilder. Frank told me that as a teenager living in New York he went to Sig Klien's gym. Frank could not afford the tuition to train at Sig's gym, so Sig told him to clean the center as an exchange for training. Frank trained there for a year before Sig gave him training routine. Adler told me that he thinks Sig was testing him to make sure that he was serious about his training. Klien told him that due to his height and long extremities that he would not be a great strongman, but he felt that he could become a great athlete if he could keep on working out hard and followed his routine. Frank asked Sig what was the secret to becoming strong. Sig's answered by telling him, "Just come." Those were two simple words, but so very true. Consistency is the key to success. Bruce Lee was quoted as saying "Long-term consistency trumps short-term intensity."

As a young bodybuilder I read about Sig, a strongman and pioneer of modern bodybuilding who is also known as the link between the old strongman and the modern bodybuilders. I never met Sig, yet he has influenced both me and my students. I'm sure he would never have imagined that his words to a teenage boy, "Just come," would be changing lives in the twenty-first century. I had a female fitness student who had never heard of Klien. She told me that she will never forget those two words, "Just come." She is now consistent in her training, rarely missing a class. As a student training in Gracie Jiu Jitsu, Tai Chi and boxing, I cherish those words. By leaving my ego at the door and not giving up, I've notice slow, but steady improvement in my Jiu Jitsu and boxing. In June 2014, I was promoted to blue belt in Gracie Jiu Jitsu. Thank you, Sig, for continuing to change lives in the 21 century.

Local Ageless Warriors

There are many local Ageless Warriors right in your neighborhood. You just don't know it because they don't look their age and they are in great shape. There are many local Ageless Warriors in great shape, men and women in their 40's, 50's, 60's 70's and beyond. As my good friend, Eric Guttman, says, "40 is the new 20!" I had some of my Ageless Warrior friends write their stories, explaining what has kept them motivated to workout and eat healthy. These are people that I admire because they are defying the odds.

You'll notice that all the Ageless Warriors I've featured are from different states and diverse occupations. They stay young by training in different modalities. The saying, "All roads lead to Rome," means there are many different routes to the same goal. There are also so many ways to get fit and stay youthful. All of the Ageless Warriors in this book have something in common. They all refuse to think old, live a healthy lifestyle and eat a healthy diet.

You'll read about my dad who built a strong body doing physical labor; my wife who is a Pilates, Fitness Kickboxing and Piloxing instructor; Eric Guttman who is a Naval Officer living in Doral who trains functionally; Pablo Zamora, a martial arts instructor from McAllen, Texas, my friend since junior high school, Jennifer Evans, and Kerry Pedlow from Laguna Beach, California who do yoga to stay youthful and surf; Sgt. John Riddle, a martial arts and fitness instructor, retired police officer and member of a SWAT Team; Frank Dimeo, my good friend who I met ten years ago at the first kettlebell instructor training workshop in Florida held at my school. Frank is incredibly strong and trains heavy at 63, and who changed his life by transforming his body and getting fit and fearless through martial arts.

Julio C. Anta, My Dad

My father, Julio Cesar Anta (June 12, 1925 - September 1, 1999), was a true Ageless Warrior. Even his name was a powerful name which is Spanish for Julius Cesar. My dad was my inspiration. He built his body functionally through hard work. In Cuba, after his father died, he had to drop out of school to support his mother and sister. He was a stevedore. He also learned to box by watching boxing matches on TV. He would go to different cities in Oriente, Cuba, boxing for money. His friends would bet money on him. He never lost a fight.

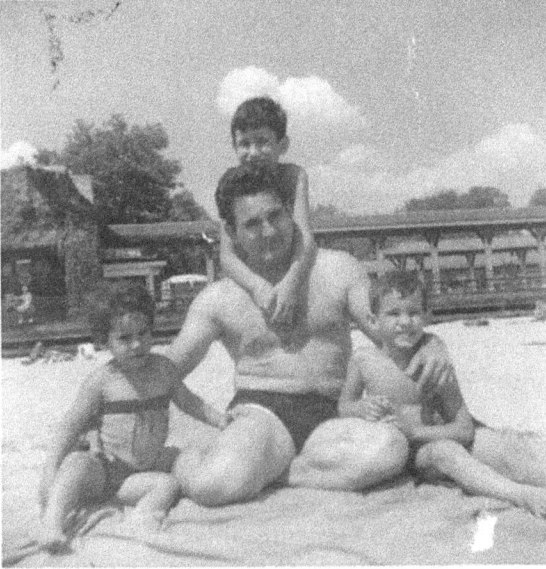

After Fidel Castro's communist regime took over Cuba, he left Cuba with my pregnant mother, my younger brother and I in pursuit of freedom.. In Yonkers, New York, he held three jobs cleaning banks, business buildings, and schools in order to support the family. He later owned a cleaning company. He took pride in cleaning the outside windows of skyscrapers. Due to my allergies and sickness, we had to relocate to Miami. In Miami, he started a new career in boat industry until he retired. He patched boats that had been in accidents, cleaned boats, and assembled boats.

When I was a teenager he would challenge me to run and he would always beat me. When I started doing karate as a teenager, we would play spar and he would always beat me with his boxing.

All his life, he worked heavy labor which kept him fit and strong. After he retired, he continued to work hard by gardening and cutting the lawn, and he always made time to workout with weights in his back yard. He also walked religiously.

My father was very disciplined. He ate healthy for five days out of the week, Monday through Friday. He would only eat desserts and junk food on Saturday and Sunday. He was a head of his time. Years later, I started reading Bill Phillips "Muscle Media 2000" magazine, 90 Days Fitness Challenge, and his book, "Body for Life," where he explained how to eat healthy six days a week and then have one cheat day. Today, people fill tires, pull ropes, use sledge hammers, lift sand bags and more to train functionally. My father built his body working hard for a living by doing similar tasks.

My father was in great shape even after an aorta valve replacement operation. He also died fit and strong. The day he passed away, he had just finished his morning walk and decided to cut the hedges. Even though, he did not have to do that since he had a younger friend who would always offer to cut his grass and do the yard work free. My dad loved gardening and being physical. While cutting the edges on a hot summer Miami day, he collapsed and died of a heart attack.

This was the hardest time of my life, since I was very close to him and admired him so much. I was blessed to have a father like him who taught me by example to work hard, have discipline, and maintain integrity. Most importantly, he taught me to be a man.

Elena Anta, My Wife

Elena was born in Port Jefferson, NY, on April 28, 1970. At 44 years old she is truly the example of the "40's being the new 20's." She is a great wife and business partner. Together we raised two healthy and fit boys, leading them by example. She is the programs director, does the accounting, and teaches Pilates, Piloxing and functional fitness at our martial arts/fitness center.

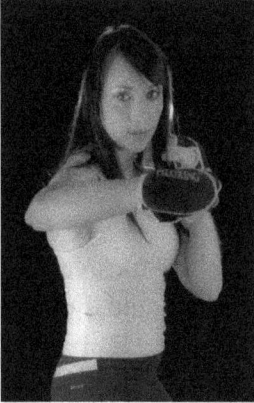

As a young girl, she danced and did some gymnastics. As a teenager, while going to high school, she had to work to help sustain her mother and younger sister after her father abandoned them. In spite of this, she still found time to do aerobic exercise.

She is a certified Pilates, Piloxing, Cardio Kickboxing, MMA Fighter Fit and an aerobics instructor. She works out with weights, yoga, jogging, Zumba, and spinning. She is also trained in women's self-defense.

Elena was at the first ever Piloxing certification in Los Angeles, California. She was the first person to be certified that did not live in California. She started the first Pilates class in North West Miami Dade County. She started the first Piloxing class in Florida. Elena and I also started the first ever fitness kickboxing class in the Doral area. Elena is a fitness pioneer in Florida bringing these programs to the City of Doral.

Even though Elena has great fitness credentials and accomplishments, I feel that her greatest accomplishment is being a great wife, inspiring and supporting me in my martial arts, fitness and business accomplishments, and also raising two successful, bright and fit young men.

Hector Arcia, My Cousin

Hector is my first cousin. His mom and my mom were sisters. We are related and share the last name of Codina. He is Hector Arcia Codina and I'm Julio Anta Codina.

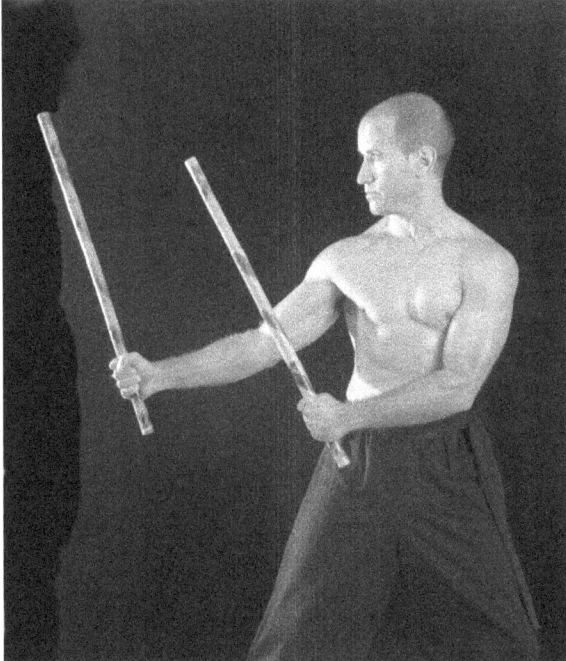

Arcia at 43 years old, stays fit by training and teaching martial arts. He teaches kung fu, Muay Thai, and fitness classes at my studio, Anta's Fitness and Self Defense.

Hector started doing martial arts at a young age due to the influence of my brothers and me. He earned his full black sash (belt) instructor under me. He is also second degree in WTF Tae Kwon Do and certified Krav Maga instructor. He is a five-time Florida state champion in Tae Kwon Do forms and sparring. Hector is a certified MMA Fighter Fit level two instructor under UFC strength and conditioning coach, Kevin Kearns.

Eric Guttman

U.S Navy

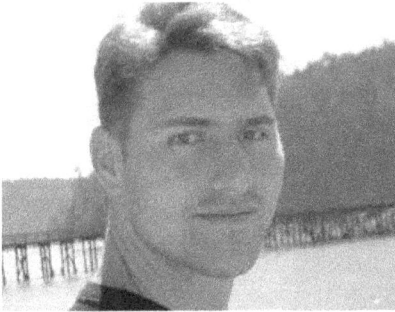

As you have read in the "Success Attracts Success" section of this book, Eric Guttman is a close friend and an important part of my inner circle. He is a 41 years old and is in excellent shape. Eric is an officer in the U.S. Navy, Krav Maga instructor, and fitness expert. When Eric got orders to report to Southern Command in Doral he called me. He was told by our mutual friend, strongman Bud Jeffries, and fitness and martial arts instructors, Darryl and Kim Brown, that when he moved to South Florida he had to meet me. Eric moved about one mile away from me. We had so much in common that we immediately became close friends. Below are Eric's own words about how he stays fit and fearless at 41.

I got interested in health and youthing (what people routinely like to call anti-aging) as well as what I currently do to remain young and vibrant. I remember it like it was yesterday, I was flying missions overland in Iraq with the U.S. Navy and after months of 18-hour days and eating galley food, which means stuff that is canned and filled with preservatives so that it can remain "viable" for long periods of time, I started to feel run down. I felt like I had hit a low point. Prior to that I followed the bodybuilding approach of training every body part once a week to achieve symmetry and I began to "eat clean." While nothing spectacular in the strength world, I had achieved "respectable" weights in the three main lifts, 405lb for the Squat, 350lbs. for the Deadlift, and 365lbs for the Bench Press. Now, while those were PRs, I trained these three lifts in the 315lb-335lb range regularly. This approach had served me well in my military career as I was able to ace the pushup and sit-up portion of my military Physical Readiness Test as well as running good times in the 1.5 mile run.

As I was contemplating my deteriorating state of health, I picked up an *Inside Kung Fu* issue in the Base Exchange we were flying out of and I saw an ad for a Qigong course. I made a DECISION to take my health back in my hands and made a mental note to order the course when I got back home, I ordered the course and started practicing regularly. I also got a book titled, "*How Long Do You Choose To Live?*" by my friend, Peter Ragnar, where he puts forth the idea of an open-ended longevity, or as I like to put it, "To Live as Long as You Can as Best as You Can!" I started changing my water and food intake and saw results within one month.

I then switched my workout philosophy from the Bodybuilding approach to the "I train my body as one unit all the time." I do not worry about leg day or chest day and I have not trained "arms" individually since 2008. I train my body as one unit so I am always symmetrical and all my workouts make me more fine-tuned with myself and my abilities. Sometimes I focus on strength and sometimes I focus more on conditioning, but when I train, I am liberated from the "looks" aspect of it and instead, I focus on ability. The correct fitness/ health pyramid should be: (1) skill in using your body which leads to (2) health which leads to (3) pleasing outward appearance because FORM FOLLOWS FUNCTION. The problem that I see in the West is that the pyramid has one dimension for the most part, which is "Look good naked" where health and skill can be sacrificed to achieve this goal. Look at all the surgeries from breast augmentations, to liposuction, to chest and butt implant for guys, as well as the slew of toxins people are willing to put in their bodies to "look" better. Just the other day I saw an article on a bodybuilder who started injecting mineral oil and alcohol in his body to "swell it up" and now he has 29 inch arms, without the STRENGTH to back it up.

A good way to track your progress is by measuring your hormones instead of your biceps. Since your hormones have a great deal to do with how you feel and perform, I started playing close attention to them and have managed to raise my testosterone naturally from an initial 585 to a 780 by modifying my exercise and eating habits along with a few supplements. By optimizing my hormones, I am able to extend my functional livelihood as well as feel young, vibrant, and alive. One of the best reasons to keep your hormones at youthful levels is because if you do so, you are ALMOST immune to disease. One of the most popular series in my blog is a four-part article titled, *"How to Get Your Hormones to Optimal Levels.*

However, with all that said, there was still a missing element which eludes most people and it eluded me for a long time. That element is RECOVERY. I really started applying this after hearing Dan Gable speak to a group and he mentioned that the key to his Olympic Gold Medals in wrestling and the champions that he coached in Iowa was due to spending as much time in recovery as they did in training. This is really the key and what most people are unwilling to do. I like how my friend and President of Agatsu, Shawn Mozen, puts it, "Everybody is willing to go into beast mode for a really tough work out and then take pictures of people collapsed on the floor drenched in sweat, but when it comes to recovery where it may involve holding an uncomfortable position, say like the bottom of a squat for a prolonged period of time, then everybody quits after ten seconds.

How do I incorporate recovery into my training? Well, one of the main ways is through joint mobility. in ways is through joint mobility. Most people allow age and decrepitude to creep in and as they age they start to stiffen up. When they stiffen up, they can't move. When they can't move their health and quality of life starts to deteriorate. Now let's look at the opposite of that, if you mobilize your body everyday so that you achieve full mobility in all your joints, and then maintain full mobility every day, then you WILL have FULL mobility for the rest of your life. My father was a Greco-Roman wrestler in Hungary and his coach told him something that has always resonated with me. He said, "If you do something every day, then every day you will be able to do it." That is why I place mobility high on the list. I do not work out every day, but I do my joint mobility every day.

Another important factor in recovery is doing cleanses. During or at the end of a training cycle, I like to do colon and liver cleanses to reset everything. In our "modern world" we are constantly bombarded with toxic chemicals in our food, air, and even from the construction materials in our homes and places of employment. Cleaning out your colon and liver will allow you to remove toxins and to absorb your nutrients better. Some people have even healed themselves of "incurable" diseases like Multiple Sclerosis and Crohn's disease by doing liver cleanses. A very interesting observation was made by Dr. Mark Hyman. He believes that there are two main causes of disease: (1) a deficiency of nutrients and/or (2) an excess of toxicity. By following a healthy diet and increasing our amount of raw and organic fruits and vegetables, we address the first cause. By performing periodic cleanses throughout our lives, we address the second cause. Another observation made by Dr. Hyman is the idea of your lifespan versus your health span. Lifespan would be the actual number of years a person lives and health span would be the number of years that person was healthy. He made the observation that in America, most people's health span is 15 years shorter than their lifespan. This means that for most Americans, their last 15 years involve decreased functionality and quality of life with increased ailments, doctor's visits, and a larger and larger portion of their income going towards medical costs instead of enjoying life.

To me the best example of lifespan and health span matching up is Jack LaLanne. He worked out all his life and had no medical conditions or infirmities. In fact he even worked out the last day he was alive and simply went to bed and did not wake up. He enjoyed a full quality of life every day and was able to depend on his body to do whatever he wanted to do. My favorite Jack LaLanne quote is, "You can do what I do if you do what I do."

Master Pablo Zamora

McAllen, Texas

I met Master Zamora in 2005 at the MAIA Martial Arts Super Show in Las Vegas. He was in line in front of me to meet David Carradine. I had known of him for a long time. When we both had long hair, people would confuse us. After we met, we became friends and noticed how much more we had in common. We are about the same height and around the same age. He was born in 1961 and I was born in 1957. We were both influenced to learn martial arts by Bruce Lee. Both of us are kung fu masters, teach Krav Maga, and Jeet Kune Do. We both were former competitive bodybuilder and were certified in Haganah F.I.G.H.T. To make things even wilder, his grandfather went to Puerto Rico from Spain and my grandfather went to Cuba from Spain. Today, we both stay fit and believe that a martial arts instructor needs to stay fit and lead by example. Here is what Master Pablo Zamora says:

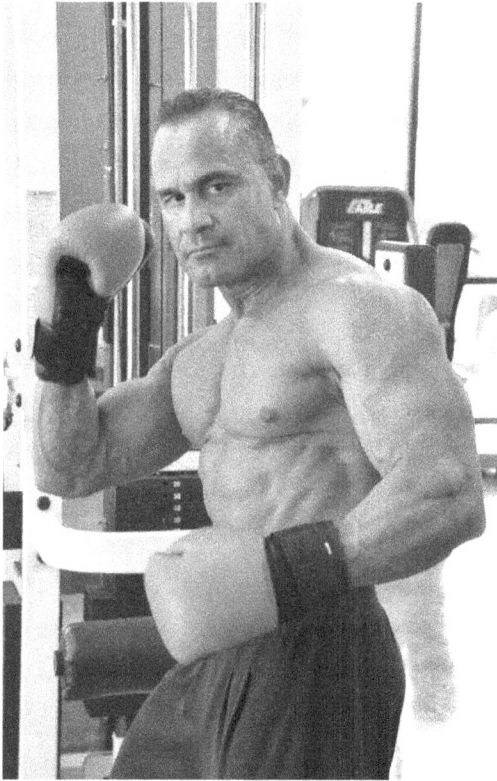

I often get asked what it is that I do to stay lean and fit over 50. My lifestyle has always been about staying in shape and functional to be able to train in my passion within the martial arts. This journey goes back about 44 years ago when I was just 8 years old. I saw Bruce Lee in *"The Green Hornet"* TV show, and it blew me away. As a kid, I loved super heroes like Superman and Batman, but Bruce Lee was in another level to me. He was "real" and his physique and ability captivated me as a kid and still does today at 52 years of age. I made it my life's quest to train myself to not only function as a warrior, but to have the skills and the physique to back it all up with, just like my childhood hero and lifelong inspiration, Bruce Lee.

I see the martial arts in a way that hopefully many others see as well. To me, a martial artist is training in the warrior ways and must commit to sharpening the skills and the body that has to execute those skills. When I see overweight and out of shape martial artists it is downright nonsense and foolishness. How can representatives of a discipline that has a history of thousands of years in creating real warriors allow this to happen to themselves. It sure makes what they say not very believable, considering that the martial arts are all about self-discipline, self-control and ultimately, self-mastery.

I made it my calling to stand-up and express my beliefs about being fit as a martial artist. This, of course, made me popular with some, but a threat to many others. The martial arts have a history that goes back about 4,000 years. This is a history of warriors training to fight for freedom and for their beliefs. This training was all about making the body tough as iron, as well as the will to go with it. Skills was one leg on the table. The other legs dealt with the strength, speed, and fitness to come out on top. This self-discipline was taught to all martial artists. The idea when one enters the martial arts is to polish that person to high gleam. This polishing can only happen by raising the bar in physical and mental training and by actually making one stronger, fitter, and highly skilled.

Knowing as child that my mission was to become a martial arts warrior like Bruce Lee. I got my father to enroll me in Karate/ Kung-Fu classes. Back in 1969, it was unusual for children to train in the martial arts here in America. But I was fortunate my teacher took me in. The training was geared for adults, so the classes were pretty tough including countless push-ups, sit-ups, deep knee bends (as they called them back then) and even pull-ups on the wall bar. Physical fitness was fifty percent of the training journey. I was excited since my teacher had Bruce Lee on the walls of the school. It was a visual reminder of why I was there training as hard as all the adults.

Many years went by and I moved and went off to another martial arts school. This was in the 1970's and the same principles applied in fitness. I was about 12 years old and was fortunate that I had three prior years of training in the martial arts. This school did not accept children, but because of my experience and ability, he accepted me. This was a dojo (martial arts school) of very high discipline. For being late or talking you got punished with 50 push-ups on the spot. I remember many classes where I did over 100 push-ups as discipline. But when I look at this today, it was the best thing that could have happened to me. As a young teen, my body began to take warrior form.

I also began to play around with weights at home and later at the local YMCA. This really got my blood boiling towards reaching higher levels in my physique and fitness. I started reading the training and nutrition in bodybuilding magazines like *Muscle Mag* and *Iron Man* and put more into wanting to develop a strong physique, while never forgetting that my goal was to be as much like Bruce Lee as local YMCA. This really got my blood boiling towards reaching higher levels in my physique and fitness. I started reading about training and nutrition in bodybuilding magazines.

I've made my living by teaching the martial arts since 1983. Around 2010, I began taking very close notice on my staff of instructors and the hundreds of students in my school. I noticed that everyone could and should be in better shape. I mean, considering that they trained daily in multiple martial art classes. Many may have been aerobically fit, but lacked the muscle shape and leanness that fit warriors are known for. We've always had a kickboxing class more for fitness, but that wasn't enough to transform people into the warrior look. I knew that they had to work their muscles more directly with resistance training, yet I didn't want to bring weights or turn my school into a gym.

It dawned on me that we could perform bodyweight exercises like I have been doing since I was a youth. I never stopped doing them even though I supplement them with weights and also with resistance bands. We have always had the students go through the basics like push-ups, crunches and squats, but not in a serious program created to burn fat and build muscle simultaneously. I listed all the bodyweight exercises that I used in my own training and created several class planners

164

to use on my team of instructors first. It was an incredible success. I put them through the training for three months and also taught them my nutritional plan. They followed it to the letter and made incredible transformations.

This got the rest of the students excited and asking questions. They wanted to know what the staff team did to get so lean and fit. I decided to open several 30-minute classes a week in what I coined, "Master Z's Warrior Fit." The training included my special report on my Master Z's Warrior Lean nutritional plan. It was an explosion of excitement and results. People loved the new training program and countless people showed their fat loss, muscle shaping results in before and after photos which we shared on Facebook. This became like a virus of motivation to family and friends of the students.

Master Z's Warrior Fit has been in my school for several years with filled classes of up to 100 training students in one single class. Of course we have to use both training floors, but the energy and excitement is tremendous. Quickly, this program became the core of what my school is all about. Assisting hundreds of people daily to get lean, fit and skilled is an incredible satisfaction. Knowing that you have everything to do with making people fit, healthy and more confident truly feels like success.

I have been consistent in resistance training (bodyweight, weights, bands, med ball) for decades. But the serious weight training with eating to get big had me at just a few pounds shy of 200 pounds. Realize that I have a small bone frame and stand about 5 feet 8 inches in height. This was a lot of muscle combined with fat. The story you read above about my staff team and students didn't begin until I myself transformed first. It took me 12 weeks to go from 198 pounds bodybuilding big to 170 pounds Warrior Fit. How did I do this? Let me explain first that I have a background in amateur bodybuilding competitions. I competed in the 80's and 90's in many shows. This gave me the experience in not just training, but in the proper nutrition to get lean while preserving muscle. It was all about getting "ripped" but holding on to as much muscle size as possible.

My 12 week transformation journey included training at the gym with weights three times a week. It also included my personal bodyweight training that was coupled along with the weights. I always complete a body part with bodyweight exercises. I may also super set (combine two or more exercises with no rest) weights with bodyweight.

Example: bench press, to decline push-ups, to flat pushups. I will do a set of bench press or chest press machine to failure. Automatically jump off and elevate my feet up on the bench and pump out as many push ups as I can do. The drop my feet parallel to the floor and push them out until I drop. I use this form of training in just about every muscle group in my body. My leg workout is quite grueling with this principle of training.

I make stretching between sets a very important part of shaping the muscles and speeding up the recuperation. The stretching helps to keep the fascia, which covers the muscles, flexible enough to allow muscle growth. Plus being a martial artist first and foremost, I do not want my muscles and joints to be too tight to move freely and quickly.

Stretching is a vital part of my Master Z's Warrior Fit training system.

 So much focus is placed on the workout and never enough on the diet. I've see this in every gym and dojo (martial arts school) I've ever trained in. I see it like this: the training is the pounding that is done with the hammer to shape the sword. But the diet is the heat that melts the steel to allow the pounding of the hammer to actually succeed in folding and shaping the sword. Bottom line is, the diet is 70% of the picture and training is 30%. Don't get me wrong, you need the training and it needs to be done correctly, but without the proper diet, the training will not give the results that transform a person from fat or skinny to warrior fit.

 It is a total science to feed the body correctly in such a way in order to burn fat while increasing muscle. This was almost unheard of decades ago when the idea was to bulk-up first and then diet down. This bulk-up and diet yo-yo was tough and didn't give the best results. But today we have the formula of eating five to six small meals a day to feed the muscles the proper amount of protein, carbohydrates and fat, while at the same time keeping the blood sugar stable and the body in fat burning mode.

 My Master Z's Warrior Lean Nutritional Plan is simple and direct. I have never been happy with diets where you had to count calories and weigh foods. My program helps you to create the most balanced meals in under 15 minutes without counting, weighing, or having to prepare fancy diet meals. Plus, you can easily eat Master Z's Warrior Lean in any restaurant. The whole idea is to learn

about our clean way of eating through our written
guide and our monthly nutritional seminars.

What I like to call "The Light At The End of the
Tunnel" is our Master Z's Warrior Fit "Cheat Meal
Time." It is the reward we get once a week on
Saturdays for a total of five hours. We get to indulge
in whatever we want to eat with no guilt or regrets.
Trust me, I can eat over 5,000 calories in that eating
time. Does it make me fat? No, not at all. Actually, I
always look my best the next couple of days after a
feeding like that. And it allows me to enjoy my
favorite bad foods without it becoming a problem in
my waistline of my health.

I had so many people contact me through email and
Facebook about my training and nutritional
program. This motivated me to expand by using
technology. I decided to have my training go global
by having a web site that will have my training
programs and nutrition available through e-learning
videos.

Jennifer Evans and Kerry Pedlow

Laguna Beach, California

I have known Jennifer Evans Kochalka since we were in junior high school and we also went to the same high school. For our first year in junior high, we went to a school with thirty of forty students called the "Neighborhood School" in Miami Springs, Florida. Jen and I found each other via Facebook. When I asked my best friend from junior high, Cort Lyber, if he remembered Jen, his answer was, "Yeah, the hot hippy chick!" Being totally honest, most people that went to school with me look old and beat up but I noticed that Jen still looked great. When I found out that her husband Kerry was 65, I was impressed and just had to have them in this book. Jennifer is also the author of *"Grand Thief Auto and Other Misdemeanors."* Here is what Jen says:

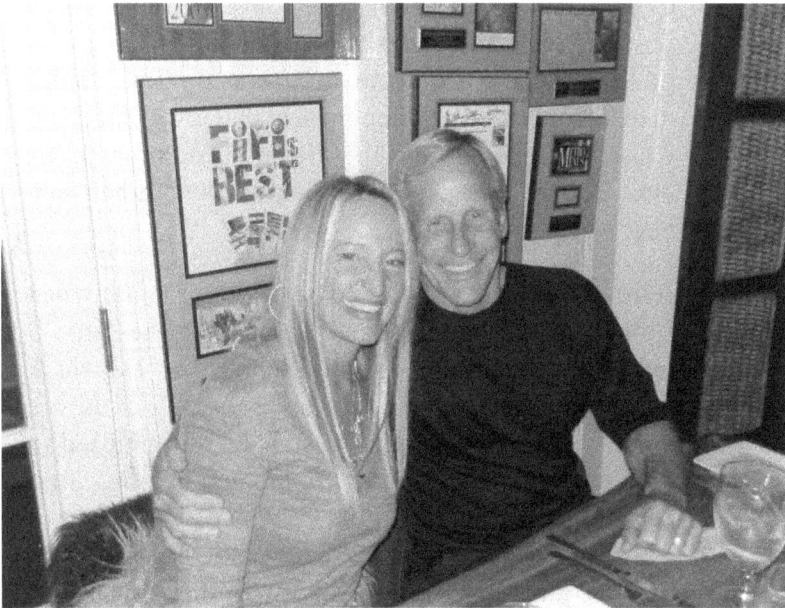

When my friend Julio Anta contacted me and asked if I'd write a chapter for his fitness book, I was thrilled. When I found out that his book features "Ageless Warriors," I thought, "Oh no, here we go again. First it's those well-meaning folks over at the AARP who are hounding me to join, and now it's Julio telling me that I'm ageless." They can't fool me. All this nice sounding verbiage is really an attempt to tell me that I'm over the hill. So why, when I wake up in the morning, do I still feel like that 12-year-old kid who used to fish tadpoles out of the local canal?

Julio, owner of Anta's Fitness and Self Defense, has been a friend since 7th grade. Although we live on opposite ends of the continent these days, he's watched the antics of my husband, Kerry, and me as we run on rugged trails, surf in the freezing Pacific Ocean, contort our bodies into extreme yoga postures in 105 degree hot yoga studios, fly trapezes in Maui, hang upside down from zip line cables made from used garden hoses in Costa Rica, all while he logs into Facebook from the comfort of his gym. Julio checks his Facebook updates in between beating up the bad guys.

Julio already knew how old I was, I'm 55, but when I told him that my husband Kerry is 65, he said, "I only hope that I can as good at 65." As the clock ticks those merciless years away, people who are much younger than we, are amazed and amused at how we manage to stay fit, active and healthy. So it is with great pride and honor that Kerry and I have enthusiastically agreed to share with Julio's readers how we have managed to stay fit all these years and have fun doing it.

I was raised by a Great Depression era father who emphasized a life of rugged individualism. As a kid in Hialeah, I watched as my dad did sit-ups, push-ups, and ran for exercise out the front door with nothing more than a pair of Ked's knock-offs and a white t-shirt and shorts. Dad would always park as far away as possible from the Grand Union grocery store entrance so that his kids had the opportunity to walk. "You don't need anything more than your own body to stay fit," he would say.

Kerry was an only child who had more energy than a high speed locomotive. His mother would worriedly rub her hands on her apron as a bottle rocket whizzed past her clothesline before demanding of Kerry's father, "Put that kid in some type of after school activity!" That was how Kerry was introduced to swimming as a competitive sport as a kid.

You may be thinking, well, those two were just born natural athletes who never had to think about fitness. Not entirely true, as I lived through the hippie generation with its emphasis on pot-smoking and Kerry lived through the 1960's when Timothy Leary was telling everyone, "Tune in, turn on, and drop out." While I'm not recommending that type of experimentation, what I've gleaned from those experiences is that we all do whatever we can to make ourselves feel better.

Make no mistake about it; "substances" do make people feel better. That's why so many people in our culture are compelled to drink a little too much fine wine, eat a little too much chocolate, take up smoking or sink into a sugar coma of Ben & Jerry's Cherry Garcia Ice Cream with extra hot fudge at the end of a rough day. Judging by the statistics of obesity, addictions and Adult Onset Diabetes in our country, I think we could all use help in how to live a healthier, fit life before those well-meaning folks at the AARP demand that we jump into a rocking chair, retire to Florida and call it a day.

Our bodies were made to move. Move it, baby! Kerry and I first met in the glassy turquoise waters of the Pacific Ocean when I was learning how to surf. I discovered that an active lifestyle is more than staying healthy. It's also a great way to meet cute guys! We surfed a wave into the sunset and have been together ever since. We all need exercise not just for our bodies, but for our minds. Exercise produces a natural high. If you've ever heard the term "runners high," I'm here to tell you that it's a very real phenomenon. When the body is stressed, an opiate-like substance called endorphin is released into the bloodstream, producing a pleasant calming effect. I decided a long time ago that if I could find a substance that would give me an opiate-like feeling without having to meet someone in a dark alley, I was going to do it. Once you discover the calming effects of endorphins, this becomes a way to replace some of the negative habits, like eating a whole bag of M & M's while sitting in a La-Z-Boy recliner watching a rerun of *Cops*. If you can find an activity that becomes a passion, then that becomes its own reward. For Kerry, it's surfing. For me, it's anything having to do with being in nature, usually on the majestic trails we have in Southern California while the delicate pink, blue and purple wild flowers are blooming. Even a gentle walk uphill will get your heart pounding, while the fresh air and sunshine rejuvenate the soul. For you, it might be something as simple as taking a walk on the beach with friends. For Kerry and I, our social life has naturally gravitated towards hanging out with others who like to surf, or hike trails, or meet at yoga class. It's a fun way to stay fit and make friends. We encourage you to find a simple activity like walking or biking—something that you can look forward too.

What about diet? I'll bet you're saying to yourself, well, those two must diet religiously! We like to abide by what we call the 80/20 rule, which means that we eat healthily 80% of the time and the other 20% of the time we pretty much eat whatever we want. If you try to restrict yourself, you are doomed to failure. It's just not realistic. The first time you pass a Dairy Queen and succumb to the Oreo Cookie Blizzard or the Brownie Earthquake Sundae, you're going to feel like a failure. We say, go ahead and have those treats once in a while and don't feel guilty about it. Just don't do it all the time. We usually eat super-healthy during the week, and then on the weekends we allow ourselves some leeway. What do I mean by super-healthy? It's pretty simple. Stay away from packaged foods as much as possible. If it's a real food that you can identify, like a vegetable or fruit, eat it. Eat organic or locally grown. Almost every town has a Farmers Market featuring fresh organic produce. But this sounds like so much work! Not really. One of the best investments we ever made was a Vita-Mix, which is a three horsepower, high speed blender. We like to start our day with fresh fruit smoothies (the internet has tons of recipes) into which we toss a handful of fresh organic baby spinach. It only takes a few minutes to put together, and we're off and running for the day.

What about food cravings? I want my Ben & Jerry's! If you like ice cream, substitute *Coconut Bliss* ice cream. It comes in yummy flavors like dark chocolate and even the plain coconut makes me feel like I'm eating something decadent. If you're handy in the kitchen, you can even make your own ice cream in the Vita-Mix. I want my potato chips! How about substituting peanuts, almonds and raisins? You can even get those in the local convenience store along with a bottle of water instead of Doritos and a Big Gulp when you're in the middle of a busy day. Our bodies grab onto every good thing we do for them and by making a few simple changes, cravings will diminish.

Kerry and I have found that there's great freedom in living a healthy lifestyle. It's easier than you think. You don't have to be a celebrity with lots of money, personal trainers, chefs and nutritionists. You don't have to be an extreme sports athlete or a fitness guru. All you need is a simple plan and a little common sense.

Not everyone wants to hang from a trapeze or zip line, but when the AARP police come looking for you, wouldn't it be nice to be able to say, no thank you? We think so.

Frank Dimeo
Sarasota, Florida

In 2004, the first kettlebell instructor that was conducted at my martial arts fitness center was where I met Frank Dimeo. There were only four people at that certification. Frank traveled 222 miles to attend the workshop. Frank and I became friends immediately. We both visit each other on occasions. I later met and got certified in Battling Ropes by the originator, John Brookfield, at John's gym. I am inspired by Frank as he succeeds and reaches personal goals yearly. His accomplishments at the age of 63 motivate me to train harder and reinforce my belief that as I age I can accomplish goals and continue to get in better shape.

> I met Julio Anta about ten years ago; he is a great martial artist, athlete, and human being. He can kick a lot guy's butts who are much younger than he is. I respect that!
> I am honored to contribute to his new book.

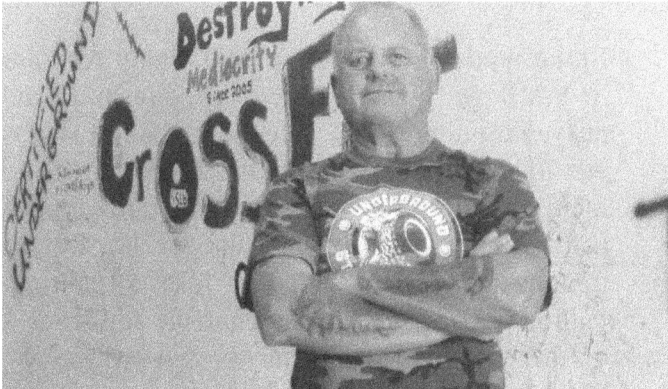

On the subject of staying fit as you age, I like to keep things very simple.

I was blessed growing up to do a lot of hard, physical work. Most of the jobs I had involved manual labor. Though it did not seem like a blessing

175

at the time, in retrospect, I was getting paid to get strong. The mindset of working hard was ingrained in me from an early age. That is one big reason I can still train hard and be healthy when many guys my age are in decline.

Right now, I am 63 years young, and I train hard 3 or 4 days a week at my gym, the Cave, in Sarasota, FL. I used to hit it hard 5 or 6 days a week, but started getting injured.

We run several training programs at the Cave: CrossFit, Underground Strength, Powerlifting, and Strongman. I believe in a strong foundation built on basic barbell lifts.
Deadlifts, squats, bench press, and shoulder press are essential for that, and are part of my training every week. I also include several bodyweight exercises that are very effective for building strength, like strict pull-ups, push-ups, squats, and lunges.

I train outdoors quite often, and highly recommend it. You'll get plenty of fresh air, sunshine, and an uneven training surface. Here I do a lot of sled work and loaded carries. Sled pulls should be done in a multi-directional manner. Pull forward, backward, and laterally; this supplements the linear type of training done with barbells. I use a variety of pulling apparatus, some anchor the tow rope high on the body, and others anchor it down around the hips. Another thing it offers is a variety of grips for pulling.

I usually bring kettlebells, dumbbells, a sandbag, a weight vest, or weight plates with me for this. Sled pushes are also effective, but I usually do those at the gym. I have several different styles of sleds for various purposes.

This is how I structure my training sessions:
I begin with about twenty minutes of
- soft tissue work/foam rolling

- joint mobility

  Next is my actual warm-up, which is another 20 to 30 minutes
- rowing, pushups, pull-ups, bodyweight squats, bear crawls, Battling Ropes

- resistance band pull-a-parts, archer pulls, face pulls

- light Olympic lifts

- finish with a specific movements mimics my training exercise

Now the work sets are done
- squat or deadlift (once a week)

- bench press or shoulder press (once a week)

- bodyweight (once a week)

- skill work (as needed) Note: basic gymnastic skills, Olympic lifts, etc.

  Accessory work/finishers
- Good mornings, dumbbell/barbell rows, weighted sit-ups, dips, resistance bands, suspension training
- I believe in training with fierce intent! Give it a legit 100% every time which brings us to rest and recovery next. When you train that had, you must recover the same way. Quality sleep is

vital, get a minimum of 7 hours every night. I can't stress the importance if this enough.

- Nutrition is next. This is also very simple, it's not rocket science. Do not follow any fad diets, period! What works for me is plenty of grass-fed beef, free-range chicken and pork, wild-caught fish, organic eggs, vegetables, fruits. I eat rice, pasta, and other ethnic foods. I don't believe in eliminating entire food groups.
- Supplementation should be kept to a minimum. A good multi-vitamin, krill or fish oil, protein, and a recovery shake should be all you need.
- I do not drink alcohol, but if you do, don't go crazy with it. Moderation is important.
- The last part is simple--no smoking or drugs, period.

I am thankful to GOD for giving me another chance to be healthy and fit after my reckless younger years. I never take even a single day for granted. Tomorrow is promised to no one. Your body is a gift, take good care of it! As the great warrior, Joshua, said, "Choose this day who you will serve. As for me and my house, we will serve the LORD."

Sgt. John Riddle (retired)
Boca Raton, Florida

I met John at his martial arts training center, Progressive Martial Arts, in 2011, when I attended Contemporary Jeet Kune Do's Edge Weapon and Law Enforcements certification. Since then John, who is 54, and I have become good friends. Here is what John says:

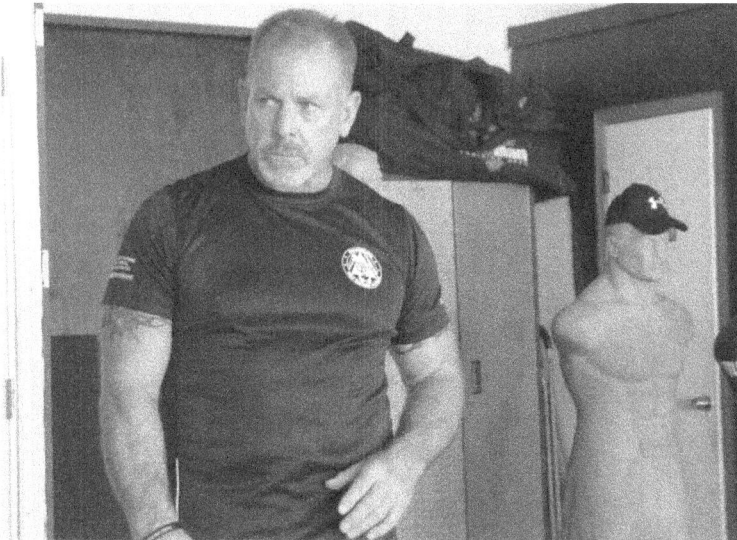

A lifetime of training pays big dividends later in life. It was back in the early 1970's when I was first introduced to weight training. I was about 16 years old. I was in high school and was interested in trying out for the football team. My weight training started paying off quickly as my strength started to increase and my body started to change and get bigger.

As years passed I continued to train with weights and entered bodybuilding competitions where I not only had a lot of fun, but I increased my weight lifting knowledge. When the time came, I entered into Military service. My weight training continued, but due to our military mission, I started to incorporate running and different types of calisthenics. This again changed my body and overall health. During this time, I was also deeply involved in martial arts. During my martial arts training, I noticed that the combination of weight training, running, and calisthenics all kicked in and came full circle to help me maintain a strong and healthy body and mind.

As I push into my mid-50's, I feel fantastic and am still pushing the limits of my body. Every day I get up and go through my routine, although different than the past, and feel that I am still getting stronger, more flexible and faster than most my age and even than most younger kids of today. Being fit and staying fit can be a long arduous effort but it pays big dividends at the end of the day!

Mike Catala

Anta's Fitness and Self Defense Martial Arts Student

Mike, as you read earlier in my book, is part of my inner circle of friends. We have become close friends since he started training at my martial arts fitness center. In two years Mike has changed his life by living the martial arts way and lifting weights. He has also led his family into a fitness lifestyle. Here is what Mike has to say:

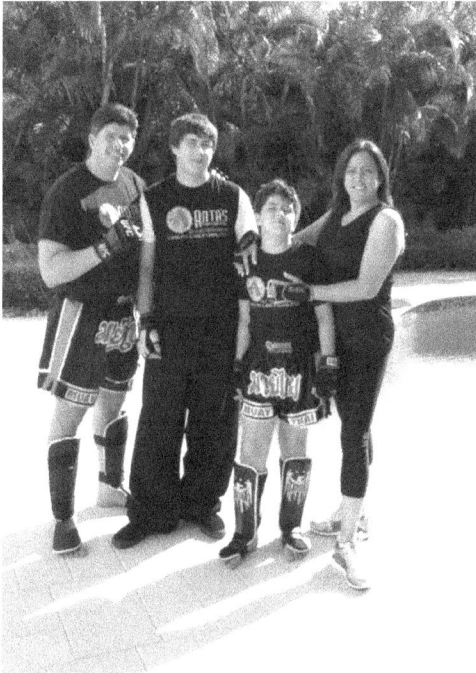

My name is Mike Catala. I am a 47-year-old working professional which, before joining Anta's School, I had never done Martial Arts. The decision to meet Mr. Anta and start training in his school was one that would create an entire paradigm shift in my life as well as my philosophy in achieving goals.

All my life I have been extremely goal-oriented as well as competitive, but, I dare say, nothing prepared me for the physical and emotional journey I was set to embark on when I decided to become a "WARRIOR".

When I joined Anta's, I picked Muay Thai kickboxing as my martial art. I was overweight, had high blood pressure, clinically depressed, and on far too many pills. I knew my life had to change first from an emotional level in order for it to transcend to the physical.

Sure enough, the first few weeks were tough. I was changing slowly, but surely. I was focused and, thanks to Mr. Anta, I wanted to become "Fit and Fearless." As the months went by, I went up in belt rank and decided to join other Martial Arts by starting in Anta's Warrior Training Program. In Anta's Warrior Training, you can train in all the martial arts that Anta teaches such as Muay Thai, Krav Maga, Jeet Kune Do, Krav Maga, and the Fitness Boot Camp. So, I started training in Kung Fu as well as Krav Maga, and even took up XFT MMA Fitness Boot Camp.

Two years later, I am now a purple belt in Muay Thai and close to achieving a lifelong dream of becoming a black belt. I see myself as an "Ageless Warrior." f Martial Arts has allowed me to really look within myself and have total control over the decisions I make in my life.

In summary, as someone who is 47, but now feels more like 27, I urge any of you to challenge yourself to discover your own warrior. Believe it or not, the emotional and physical journey will lead you to discover there are no limits to what you can achieve. To quote the Marines "Failure is not an Option"

About the Author

Julio Anta is the video author of *"The Art of Fighting Without Fighting," "Anti-Bullying(tm),"* and *"Shaolin Physical Conditioning."* He co-owns with his wife, Elena, one of Florida's most successful martial arts and fitness centers, fulfilling his childhood dreams. His center is located in Doral, a suburb of Miami, Florida.

To keep up with his latest news you can go to his blog:
www.martialartsandfitness.typepad.com
You can also log on to his websites:
www.antamartialarts.com
www.miamikettlebell.com
www.artoffightingwithoutfighting.com
www.doralkravmaga.com,
www.floridajeetkunedo.com
www.doralfitnesschallenge.com
You can also find him and his center on most social media sites.

Martial Arts and Fitness Certifications:
Hung Gar Kung Fu Master
International Association of Krav Maga Level 2 Instructor
C.O.R.E Krav Maga Instructor
KMMA Krav Maga Martial Arts Instructor
Jeet Kune Do Athletic Association Coach One Instructor
Paul Vunak's Progressive Fighting System Jeet Kune Do Phase One Instructor
Progressive Fighting System Edge Weapon Instructor
Progressive Fighting System Law Enforcement Instructor
Military JKD & SPECOPS Kali certified
Muay Thai Instructor (Trans Muay Thai Association) Level 3 Kru Instructor
Haganah F.I.G.H.T. (Fierce Israeli Guerrilla Hand to hand Tactics) Instructor
SABER Edge Weapons Combative's Instructor
Gracie Jiu Jitsu blue belt under Valenti Brothers Jiu Jitsu

Burn with Kearns MMA Fighter Fit Level 3 Instructor
Action Strength Instructor
Battling Ropes Instructor
Fitness Kickboxing Instructor
Kardio Karate Instructor
ISSA Fitness Instructor (Personal Trainer)
HKC Kettlebell Certification
Mike Mahler Level 1 Kettlebell Workshop
ECF (Elite Combat Fitness) Instructor
Elite Kettlebell Instructor
Kettlebell Concepts Kettlebell Instructor
IYCA (International Youth Conditioning Association) Youth
Fitness Specialist
ISKA MMA Referee
National Security Agency certified Child Safety Agent
Dr. Terrence Webster-Doyle Martial Arts for Peace Bully
Buster instructor
ACMA (American Council of Martial Arts) certified Martial
Arts Instructor by the Copper Institute
Dr Ben Lerner's Maximized Living Mentor
ICS Fitness and Nutrition Instructor
Pilates Physical Minds Institute
All American Pilates

Awards/Organizations:

2013-2014 Best of Doral
-2012 City of Doral Proclamation Anta's Art of Fighting
without Fighting Anti-Bullying Day
-2012 Miami-Dade County Proclamation Anta's Art of Fighting
without Fighting Anti-Bullying Day
-2012 Best of City Search
-2011-2014 PMA (Professional Martial Arts Association) Best
School in Doral
-2010 Doral 5K 3rd Place Winner
-2009 Best of Doral Martial Arts Award
-2009-2011 Century Martial Arts Mark of Excellence Award
-2006 United States Martial Arts Hall of Fame Kung Fu Master

-2006 World Martial Arts Union Hall of Fame Life Achievements
-2006 Miami Dade County Certificate of Appreciation
-2006 Captain of the runners up in the South Florida Dragon Boat Festival 250 Meter Kung Fu Cup
-2005 EFC Black Belt Schools "Outstanding Martial Arts School"
-2005 EFC Black Belt Schools "Hero Award"
-2005 Proclamation "Anta's Fitness and Self Defense Day" City of Doral
-2004 Miami Dade County "Martial Arts Excellence Award"
-2003 Florida Martial Arts Hall of Fame "Instructor of the Year"
-1998 Florida PBA Certificate of Appreciation
-1983 2nd runner up Jr. Florida Bodybuilding Championships
-1983 2nd runner up Miami Bodybuilding Championship

Julio has been a guest on Univision's Control, Despierta America, Noticias 23, Al Amanecer, Primer Impacto, mun2 Fuzion, Telefutura's Veredicto Final, CBS 4 News, WPLG TV 10 News on ABC, Channel 7 Fox News, CV Network, Telefutura, Galavision, Today in South Florida, Telemundo's News, Buenos Dias, Al Rojo Vivo, TVC's Una Hora Contigo, Ch 41 America TeVe News, Quiereme Descalsi, Miami Contigo, Show de Fernando, Pax's Aleph TeVe, TBN Joy in our Town, UMTV News, Telemundo's Al Rojo Vivo, Levántate, Un Nuevo Día, Titulares Y Mas, Deco Drive, Fuzion DNA and numerous other TV shows.

Today he writes a column for Ciudad Doral newspaper. Mr. Anta wrote a column for the Doral Tribune for 13 years. He also had a column in Doral Planet and Doral Lifestyle magazines. His articles have been published in Tae Kwon Do Times, Journal of Asian Martial Arts, Martial Arts Professional, Dragon Boat World, Fytness Fanatiks, NAPMA Now, and Trumpeter Magazine

Authors other Resources

Anta's Art of Fighting Without Fighting Anti-Bullying

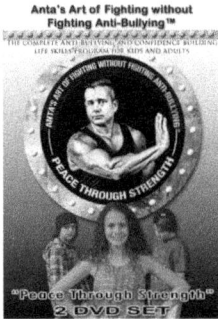 A complete Anti-Bullying program for kids, teens and adults. This program was inspired by Bruce Lee and President Ronald Reagan. You'll hear stories of my experience with bullies as a child and as an adult. Great video for school teachers, martial arts instructors, church groups and anyone the works with kids.
Downloadable $39.99, 2 DVD Set $49.99

Anta's Shaolin Physical Conditioning

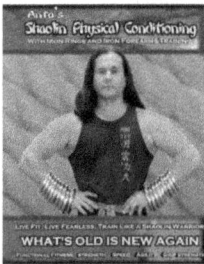 My first video. Yeah, that's me with the long hair. It covers Shaolin Kung Fu fitness, Iron Ring training, hard Qi Gong, forearm training and bodyweight exercise. Train like a Shaolin Warrior.
Downloadable $29.99
DVD $39.99

King Moringa Pills

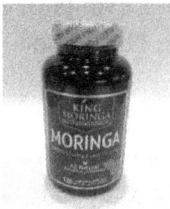 This is the Moringa pills that I use and recommend. A bottle will last you one month. To get the full effects of Moringa you need to use it continuously for three months.
1 bottle for $25, 2 for $40

To order log on to http://www.AntaMartialArts.com or call Anta's Fitness and Self Defense at 305 599-3649

.

www.ingramcontent.com/pod-product-compliance
Lightning Source LLC
Chambersburg PA
CBHW031511270326
41930CB00006B/363